DISGUSTING
THINGS

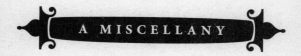

A MISCELLANY

DISGUSTING THINGS

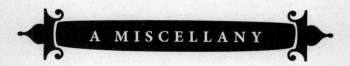

A MISCELLANY

Don Voorhees

A Perigee Book

A PERIGEE BOOK
Published by the Penguin Group
Penguin Group (USA) Inc.
375 Hudson Street, New York, New York 10014, USA

Penguin Group (Canada), 90 Eglinton Avenue East, Suite 700, Toronto, Ontario
M4P 2Y3, Canada (a division of Pearson Penguin Canada Inc.) • Penguin Books
Ltd., 80 Strand, London WC2R 0RL, England • Penguin Group Ireland, 25 St.
Stephen's Green, Dublin 2, Ireland (a division of Penguin Books Ltd.) • Penguin
Group (Australia), 250 Camberwell Road, Camberwell, Victoria 3124, Australia
(a division of Pearson Australia Group Pty. Ltd.) • Penguin Books India Pvt. Ltd.,
11 Community Centre, Panchsheel Park, New Delhi—110 017, India • Penguin
Group (NZ), 67 Apollo Drive, Rosedale, North Shore 0632, New Zealand (a division
of Pearson New Zealand Ltd.) • Penguin Books (South Africa) (Pty.) Ltd., 24 Sturdee
Avenue, Rosebank, Johannesburg 2196, South Africa

Penguin Books Ltd., Registered Offices: 80 Strand, London WC2R 0RL, England

While the author has made every effort to provide accurate telephone numbers and
Internet addresses at the time of publication, neither the publisher nor the author
assumes any responsibility for errors, or for changes that occur after publication.
Further, the publisher does not have any control over and does not assume any
responsibility for author or third-party websites or their content.

First edition: August 2008

Library of Congress Cataloging-in-Publication Data

Voorhees, Don.
    Disgusting things : a miscellany / Don Voorhees.— 1st ed.
        p. cm.
    Includes bibliographical references.
    ISBN 978-0-399-53433-1
    1. Body fluids.   2. Food.   3. Animals.   4. Aversive stimuli.   I. Title.
    QP90.5.V67 2008
    612'.01522—dc22   2008000736

PRINTED IN THE UNITED STATES OF AMERICA

10   9   8   7   6   5   4   3   2   1

Most Perigee books are available at special quantity discounts for bulk purchases for
sales promotions, premiums, fund-raising, or educational use. Special books, or book
excerpts, can also be created to fit specific needs. For details, write: Special Markets,
Penguin Group (USA) Inc., 375 Hudson Street, New York, New York 10014.

This book is dedicated in memory of my father,
who would have gotten a real kick out of it.

ACKNOWLEDGMENTS

Thanks to my literary agent, Janet Rosen, for her great enthusiasm and for finding a wonderful home for this book at Penguin. Thanks to my editor, Meg Leder, who had the vision for this project before I did and whose expert guidance and insights are greatly appreciated. Also, thanks to her intern Brian Schacter for all his hard work. Thanks to Ben Gibson for designing a really creepy cover. Thanks to Jennifer Eck and Candace B. Levy for a very thorough, professional copyedit. Finally, thanks to my wife and kids, who are always supportive of my writing and understand when I disappear into the den for hours on end to research and peck away on my laptop.

CONTENTS

INTRODUCTION: WHY DO CERTAIN THINGS DISGUST YOU?

Let's face it, life is gross. We don't find rocks or stars disgusting, and rarely plants. By definition, for something to be repulsive, it almost has to involve people, animals, or food. Different folks are disgusted by different things. Saliva makes some people gag, while others walk around expectorating (spitting) all day long. Certain sounds, sights, smells, and tastes seem to be universally abhorred. The sound and smell of someone vomiting, the sight of puss-oozing wounds, and corpses come immediately to mind. Disgust is common to all cultures. It can lower your blood pressure and make you nauseous, shudder, or take evasive action.

In general, things that can make us ill, we find disgusting. In evolutionary terms, this is an innate reaction designed to protect us from harm. For example, the vast majority of us are repelled by the bodily excretions and secretions of others; this is a good thing because they contain pathogens that can enter our bodies and make us sick. Women tend to feel disgust more easily than men because they play the double role of protecting themselves *and* their offspring—or so researchers say. By the same reasoning, as we grow older, we are less easily disgusted because our chances of having children are not as great. Strangers are more disgusting because they may carry germs that we are not familiar with. If you are buying any of these theories, keep in mind being grossed out is just nature's way of helping to keep you healthy.

Oddly enough, many of us find a perverse pleasure and fascination in gross things. It's like when you pull an old carton of milk out of the fridge that you know has gone bad, yet you are still compelled to sniff it. Beware, this book is filled with far more cringe-worthy things than sour milk. Within these pages I have compiled as much deliciously disgusting trivia as possible, which leads us to the first chapter.

Proceed at your own risk.

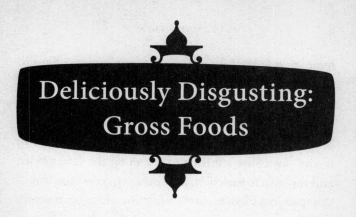

Deliciously Disgusting: Gross Foods

Some forms of disgust are learned, not innate. Take food for example. There are great cultural differences found around the world. Many people are uncomfortable or even repulsed by foods that are foreign to them. While some of us may find monkey brains disgusting, others are repelled by the thought of a beef patty covered in cheese. This chapter looks at extreme foods from near and far, in all their stomach-turning glory.

Where do they drink frog juice?

This may sound like a bad Kermit the Frog joke, but folks in Peru take frog juice quite seriously. Nicknamed "Peruvian Viagra," this nasty concoction is believed by Andean cultures to be an aphrodisiac and to cure asthma, bronchitis, and sluggishness. Restaurants in Lima specialize in steaming hot mugs of frog juice, and many people treat it as their morning cup of coffee. So what exactly is this stuff?

As its name implies, it's blended frogs. Frogs are kept in aquariums at restaurants; and to make frog juice, the cook selects a frog and then bangs on its head until it dies. Two slits are then made along the frog's belly, and the skin is peeled off as if husking corn. The frog is dropped in a blender containing hot white-bean broth, honey, aloe vera, and maca (a root thought to increase stamina and libido); and the mix is puréed. The resultant hot froth is strained and served up like a disgusting frog milkshake. It stings the throat, but it's a real bargain at about 90 cents a cup.

What traditional alcoholic beverage is made with human saliva?

If you ever get down Ecuador way, you've got to try chicha. It is the staple drink of the Achuar tribe. The women there *really* put themselves into this beverage. It is made with a little love and a lot of spit. That's right! The ladies chew on cooked yucca plant and spit the macerated glop into a bowl and leave it there to ferment into chicha. Locals love the stuff and are proud to serve it to houseguests, who are obliged to drink. However, outsiders have a hard time stomaching chicha, which smells like bread and vinegar and tastes just like, you guessed it, spit. (Talk about a mouthwatering beverage.)

Traditional chicha can also be found in isolated areas of Peru and Bolivia. The indigenous peoples of South and Central America have been fermenting a variety of crops with their saliva for thousands of years. An Inca favorite was a chicha beer made from maize (corn) and saliva. Called *chicha de jora*, it has an alcohol content of between 1 and 3 percent. It has a milky, pale yellow color and a flavor akin to hard cider with a sour aftertaste. Quinoa, carob seeds, fruits, and vegetables are also fermented this way.

What is the most foul-tasting beverage?

This is a judgment call, but it's probably an alcoholic beverage called pruno concocted by the inmates of the California penal system. Prisoners are deprived of most of life's pleasures, including alcohol. With nothing but time on their hands, they tend to come up with some pretty ingenious ways to make life behind bars more bearable, one being pruno. There are no prunes in pruno, but there's plenty of gross. To make your own pruno, follow this simple procedure:

1. Take 10 peeled oranges and an 8½-ounce can of fruit cocktail and dump them into a large resealable plastic food bag.
2. Mash them together furiously.
3. Now add 16 ounces of hot tap water.

4. Next, take the bag of warm fruit slop and wrap it up in a towel to hide it from the guards or just to keep it warm to speed fermentation.

5. After 48 hours, you will have a gas-inflated bag of fermented mush that smells like nasty bread dough gone wrong.

6. To really get the fermentation going, it's time to add something sweet; six packets of ketchup and about 50 sugar cubes should do the trick.

7. Smoosh ingredients around until you have a bag of red slime.

8. Now soak the bag in hot water for 30 minutes to kick-start fermentation.

9. Rewrap in towel and hide from the guards, or your mother, for 3 days, reheating once a day.

10. Open occasionally to release gas buildup and avoid having to deal with a messy pruno explosion.

11. Spoon out or strain the bits of fruit that still remain intact, leaving just the liquid.

You now have a plastic bag of what looks and smells like vomit, according to aficionados (i.e., inmates). Those white splotches floating around in your pruno are mold, which only adds to the charm of the drink. Done correctly, this recipe will yield about 2 pints of pruno with up to a 14 percent alcohol content, just enough for you and your sweetheart, or prison friend, to get a little hammered and a lot nauseous.

In 2002, California prisons began banning oranges, raisins, and sugar packets to reduce the amount of pruno produced. Undeterred, the ever-resourceful inmates have switched to other ingredients, like sauerkraut and orange juice.

What coffee is made from turds?

This may seem like one of those questions that must be made up, but read on. Not only does such coffee exist but it is one of the most expensive in the world, selling for as much as $300 a pound.

The common palm civet (*Paradoxurus hermaphrodites*) is a Southeast Asian cat-like omnivore with a taste for coffee beans. A relative of the raccoon, this 4- to 11-pound creature spends most of its time in the trees, emerging at night to feed on small mammals, insects, and fruits. A common resident of coffee plantations, the palm civet dines heavily on coffee cherries (the ripe fruit the coffee bean comes from).

Far from being a pest, these little guys are welcome guests at the coffee plantations of the Philippines, Indonesia, and Vietnam. Palm civets digest only the outer pulpy part of the fruit. The coffee beans themselves pass through their digestive systems and are excreted by the animals. Because the civets repeatedly poop in piles and at the same spots, their droppings are easily collected.

Why would anyone want to collect civet dung? Because the beans found therein can be roasted and brewed into what's known as *kopi luwak*—civet coffee. Many believe it to be the world's finest because the civets select and eat only the ripest coffee cherries. The beans are slightly fermented during their travels through the civet's gastrointestinal tract. Chemical analyses show these beans have fewer of the proteins that can cause bitterness, and different volatile compounds responsible for flavor and aroma, than do unfermented beans.

Annual global supply is only about 600 to 700 pounds, which accounts for the coffee's price. So what does coffee that came out of a civet's rear end taste like? Think *gamy*.

Why does orange juice taste funny after you brush your teeth?

There's nothing like the sweet, fresh taste of orange juice first thing in the morning. If you don't wait a little while after brushing your teeth, however, the lingering toothpaste in your mouth will foul the taste of your orange juice.

There is nothing wrong with your toothpaste or your orange juice. The two just don't mix well in your mouth. Most toothpastes contain a chemical foaming agent called sodium lauryl sulfate (SLS). Any leftover SLS in your mouth will react with the natural acids in the orange juice, reducing its sweetness and allowing the bitter notes in the juice to stand out. Thankfully, SLS dissipates quickly, and in a few minutes your OJ can be fully enjoyed again.

Why don't Westerners eat horse meat?

Extremely nutritious, low in fat, high in protein, and packed with vitamins and iron, horse meat is very tender and slightly sweet, tasting something like a cross between beef and venison. Although some people don't care for its flavor, this is not the reason Americans don't eat equine burgers. The Western world's taboo on eating horse meat goes back to at least the eighth century.

In ancient Europe, pagans believed that supernatural spirits resided in horses. They ritually sacrificed horses and consumed their flesh in sacred ceremonies. This practice didn't sit too well with the early Christian church. In 732 CE, Pope Gregory III (reigned 731–741) banned the eating of horses as an unclean and evil act. While the pope's proclamation greatly reduced the number of horse steaks gracing the Dark Age dinner table, the ritual sacrifice of equines persisted well into the second millennium. Horses were killed at the funerals of both King John of England in 1216 and Holy Roman Emperor Karl IV in 1378.

Jewish and Islamic cultures have never eaten horse. Under Mosaic law, the horse is considered ritually unclean because it is not cloven hoofed and cud chewing.

Many countries don't share the American abhorrence of eating horse flesh. It is a favored food in Kazakhstan and other Central Asian nations as well as in Quebec and some European countries. Horse meat is particularly popular in France and Belgium and to a lesser extent in Spain, Italy, Germany, Austria, Switzerland, and the Netherlands.

Most Westerners today don't avoid horse meat for religious reasons but for aesthetic ones. As with dog meat and cat meat, many people are repulsed by eating any animal that also is kept as a pet. (Lucky for Mister Ed.)

In times of hardship, however, even Americans have condescended to eating "lowly" horse meat. During World War II, the state of New Jersey legalized its sale to alleviate a beef shortage. At the end of the war, the ban on horse meat was reinstated. In the early 1970s, toward the end of Richard Nixon's second term, the price of beef skyrocketed and some Americans tried horse meat for the first time (This scenario was hilariously illustrated in an episode of the hit television show of the time *All in the Family,* where Michael and Gloria got some horse meat that Edith unwittingly served to Archie, who ate it with gusto.)

Although Americans don't eat much horse meat, it may surprise you to learn that the country raises around 50,000 horses a year to be slaughtered for consumption elsewhere! Most of this meat goes to Mexico, Europe, and Japan. The Japanese enjoy a dish called *sakura,* which is a horse meat sashimi (sliced raw horse meat). Some of it is used to feed carnivores in zoos. In fact, it is believed that 1986 Kentucky Derby winner and 1987 Horse of the Year Ferdinand, having outlived his usefulness as a stud horse in Japan, was slaughtered in 2003 and sold as pet food. Many countries, such as

China, Mexico, Argentina, Italy, and Kazakhstan, produce hundreds of thousands of tons of horse meat every year.

Because horses aren't susceptible to mad cow disease, horse meat is gaining in popularity around the world. Some animal lovers (living animal lovers, that is) prefer horse meat over beef because the horses, in some countries, are killed in a more humane way than are mass-produced cattle. The horses are taken out into an open space, given some food, and shot in the head with a metal bolt. We should all meet such a "humane" end.

What is liquid cat?

If you found the thought of eating horses to be repugnant, this one will really repulse you. Many peoples eat cats and dogs. Cats are eaten in fewer countries than are dogs. The folks of Guangdong Province in China go for cat in a big way. Stray felines are routinely collected off the streets and many owned pets are stolen to meet the demand for cat meat. The *South China Morning Post* reported in 2002 that close to 10,000 cats a day are rounded up off the streets of Beijing for the dinner table.[1] The majority are sold to restaurants.

The most offensive thing to Westerners concerned with feline rights in China is not just the fact that cats are eaten but how they are prepared (squeamish cat lovers may wish to avoid the rest of this entry). Although some of the kitties destined for the dinner table are killed in the market, usually by strangulation, most are dispatched at the restaurant. Being fanatics for fresh food, the Chinese cooks throw the live cats into pots of boiling water to make them easier to skin.

Korean cooks quickly parboil living cats for *Goyangitan,* a traditional remedy and health food. Koreans believe that the adrenaline rush the cats experience creates a more tasty and potent meat. Quite often the cats are boiled so quickly that they are still semiconscious and twitching when skinned!

Thankfully, the sale of cat meat is illegal in the United States; however, there are websites devoted to the best ways to skin and eat a cat, so it may be going on out there behind closed doors. Apparently, there really *is* more than one way to skin a cat.

What country raises Saint Bernards for food?

The Chinese just *love* Saint Bernards—as food, that is. Dogs are eaten in several Asian countries, and China in particular seems to have developed a taste for Saint Bernards. The breed is imported from Switzerland and inbred or bred with mutts raised specifically for this purpose. Saint Bernards are favored because they quickly grow to be very large, which makes the breeders lots of money, four times as much as can be made raising pigs or chickens. The meat is more tender than other dog meat, which can be tough to chew.

The Chinese also have a fondness for the black-tongued Chow Chow. In fact, the term *chow chow* is Chinese slang for anything edible. The Chinese believe that the bluer the dog's tongue, the sweeter the meat will be.

There are restaurants in Beijing that specialize in dog dishes. One is called the Gourou Wang, meaning "Dog Food King" (is this anything like Burger King?). Menu offerings include dog ribs, stewed dog meat with soy sauce, stewed paws and tail with ginseng, and boiled dog meat soup.

North Koreans, like their neighbors to the west, have a yen for dog. In the early 1980s, as North Korea was suffering chronic food shortages, Kim Il Sung, the country's first dictator, hailed dog meat's nutritional value. One of the country's favorite dishes is *dangogi-jang,* which means "dog meat soup"; another is canine intestines. Dog meat became a luxury food after the famines of the mid-1990s. The country is now so poor that even the dogs are emaciated, which has cut down on the trade of dogs from North Korea into China.

In South Korea, where food is plentiful, people enjoy a dog dish known as *boshintang,* or "health soup." Authorities temporarily banned the sale of dog meat while hosting the 1988 Olympics, for fear of adverse international publicity. But don't expect the Westminster Kennel Club show in South Korea anytime soon.

Who on Earth eats partially developed duck embryos out of the egg?

Balut is the hard-boiled egg from hell (at least to Westerners). It is a popular Filipino snack that is sold by street vendors in the same way hot dogs are on city streets in America. Although there are some gross ingredients in hot dogs (that's another story), balut will turn the stomach of even the most adventurous Western diner. So what the heck is it?

Balut doesn't fit into any convenient category. It falls somewhere between an egg and a duck, combining the worst aspects of both. It's a fertilized duck egg with a half-developed embryo inside. The 17- to 20-day-old fetus is not quite old enough to have a beak and feathers, and its bones are still quite soft. These fertilized eggs are kept warm in the sun until they are ready to be cooked and eaten. Vendors then sell them out of buckets of warm sand. These hideous embryo eggs are cracked open and served with a pinch of coarse salt.

The Vietnamese like their balut a little more developed, so that the little duckling is more recognizable, with half-formed feathers and bones that are nice and crunchy. Of course, it's just a matter of taste. You will, however, need to pick the feathers out of your teeth.

Where do they eat cobra hearts?

This entry is hands down the most deliciously disgusting food item in the book. There are restaurants in Vietnam that serve still-beating cobra heart. The unfortunate snake is brought out to your table. A pair of scissors is used to cut open the underside of the slithering serpent. Your waiter then pushes his fingers into the cobra and literally rips its heart out. The still-pulsating organ is immediately put in a dish and served up. It is meant to be swallowed whole, still twitching as it slides down your throat, and can be chased with a glass of cobra blood. The more squeamish diner may drop the heart into a glass of rice wine before swallowing.

If you think this *sounds* gross, you should *see* it in action.[2] Anthony Bourdain, the TV food adventurer, takes the heart right down with gusto on his show *No Reservations*. You can also go online[3] to see Bourdain eating this dish as well as balut (see page 12)—if you dare. Be prepared to gag.

Who eats placentas?

Most mammal species, including all primates (except most humans, that is), eat placentas. Females who have just given birth derive nutrition from the placenta, which saves them having to leave their newborn to seek food. And, yes, incredibly, some people eat them, too! There are doctors and midwifes who preach that the eating of one's placenta has many health benefits, including easing postpartum depression and postpartum hemorrhage. Eating one's own placenta doesn't pose any health risks per se, but be careful about eating someone else's. You never know what blood diseases you may pick up.

So what does placenta taste like? No, not chicken, but beef. It has a springy texture, similar to the heart, which is something else most people will never eat.

How does one prepare it? Placenta can be substituted for meat in any number of dishes, such as lasagna, pizza, or spaghetti. It can also be dehydrated and used as a powder. However you prepare placenta, make sure to remove the membranes and umbilical cord first.

The most popular method of preparing placenta is to dry and powder it. The desiccated placenta can be sprinkled on cereal, mixed in drinks, or added to your favorite recipes. Some women even fill Gelcaps with their powdered placenta to take as a daily supplement.

Do people really eat live monkey brains?

One of the most disgusting movie scenes in recent memory is the banquet sequence in *Indiana Jones and the Temple of Doom,* in which they eat chilled monkey brains. Many peoples do indeed eat monkey brains. There is debate, however, about whether the practice of eating live monkey brains really exists today. According to a 1998 report in the *Apple Daily,* a Hong Kong newspaper, some remote Chinese village inns still cater to live-monkey-brain enthusiasts.[4] In the south-western Guangxi Zhuangzu Province, near the border with Vietnam, gourmets can buy monkeys at markets and take them to certain restaurants for their dining pleasure.

How does one eat live monkey brains? Right out of the head of a live monkey, of course. Traditionally, the monkey was secured under a special table that had a hole in the top for the monkey's head to stick out. The monkey's mouth was then sealed to prevent him or her from screaming, which can be a bit of a distraction for the diner. The top of the head was shaved and the skull cut open.

Deemed too cruel for modern sensibilities, the dining experience is a little different today. The unfortunate primate is first forced to drink enough rice wine to get good and inebriated. Then, after the monkey is passed out drunk, his or her head is opened and the brains are scooped out with spoons while the blood vessels are still visibly pulsing away. Seasonings such as pickled ginger, chili pepper, fried peanuts, and cilantro add flavor to this otherwise bland dish. Now that's "good eats!" (as Alton Brown would say).

After the brains are eaten, the rest of the monkey parts go into other dishes. The paws and muscles make a good stock and the eyeballs can go into monkey soup. (In some Arab and North African countries, people savor stuffed sheep's eyeballs.)

Technically, the eating of monkeys is illegal around

the world, but gourmets in China, Indonesia, and the Philippines keep the dish alive.

Are squirrel brains bad for you?

Have you ever eaten squirrel brains? No? Well, here's one more reason not to—they may drive you mad, or even kill you!

Squirrel brains have long been a regional delicacy in rural Kentucky and other parts of the American South, such as Alabama, Mississippi, and West Virginia. Folks in western Kentucky eat either squirrel meat or brains, not both, depending on local tradition. Those who eat the meat generally prepare it with vegetables in a stew called burgoo. Roadkill squirrels are often thrown into the pot.

Those folks who prefer squirrel brains have their own ritual. A severed squirrel head is often given to the family matriarch as a gift by a visitor. She will shave the fur off the top and fry it whole. When done, the skull is cracked open and the brains sucked out. Sometimes, the walnut-size brains are scooped out of the skull first and scrambled up with white gravy or eggs for a yummy Sunday brunch!

Doctors now warn against eating squirrel brains because they may carry a variant of mad cow disease called Creutzfeldt-Jakob disease, which can be fatal to humans. Roadkill squirrels are more likely to be infected than ones shot hunting because the disease makes the animals more likely to stagger onto the road-way. People infected with Creutzfeldt-Jakob disease will develop a serious case of the staggers, lose their wits, and probably end up dead. One hell of a price to pay to eat squirrel brains.

What states let you eat your roadkill?

Yes, there are states where collecting your roadkill is not only legal but encouraged. The West Virginia state leg-islature passed a law in 1998 allowing motorists to keep their roadkill; residents can take it home and eat it, so long as they report their windfall to the state authorities within 12 hours. This saves the highway division the time and expense of picking up all those dead critters. (Some states, however, seem to save the time and money by just letting the carcasses rot away on the shoulder of the highway.)

About 1.5 million deer are hit by cars every year in the Untied States. Can you guess the number one deer-kill state? It's Pennsylvania, followed by Michigan and Illinois. In Pennsylvania, where over 40,000 whitetails a year are creamed by cars, it's legal to claim a deer you hit. You must be a Pennsylvania resident and you need to report it to the game commission within 24 hours to do so. If you don't want it, another passing Pennsylva-nia driver may just take it.

If you are interested in sampling some tasty road-kill dishes but don't fancy scraping a flattened critter up off he interstate, check out the Roadkill Cookoff in Marlinton, West Virginia. It was inaugurated to celebrate that state's roadkill legislation. Held annually in September, the cookoff includes such folksy fare as Tire Tread Tortillas, Thumper Meets Bumper, and Deer on a Stick.

What are prairie oysters?

Prairie oysters may be the most repulsive of all regional American food. Also known as Rocky Mountain oysters, they are pan-fried bull testicles.

When male calves are branded, they are also castrated and become what are known as steers. They have their balls removed to make them meatier and more sedate. Not ones to waste anything, cowboys peeled and washed the testicles, rolled them in flour and butter, and fried them up. These oysters are still considered to be a delicacy. Bull testicles can also be served deep-fried, marinated, or cut into thin slices. Deep-fried prairie oysters have the taste and texture of calamari.

Each year in the spring and fall, there are several testicle festivals (say that five times fast) held in Montana and one in Calgary, Alberta, in Canada. At the one in Clinton, Montana, connoisseurs gobble up 2.5 tons of bulls' balls. (Speaking of gobbling, the Turkey Testicle Festival is held every October in Byron, Illinois.) If you can't make it to one of the festivals, you can order prairie oysters at numerous restaurants in Montana, Idaho, and Kansas.

What are sweetbreads?

Well, sweetbreads certainly aren't bread, and they certainly aren't sweet; but they definitely are gross. Sweetbreads are the thymus glands of veal, young beef, lamb, and pork. There are two thymus glands: a large, round one near the heart and a smaller, elongated one in the throat. The heart sweetbread is more desirable and expensive because of its delicate flavor and firmer, creamier texture. The best sweetbreads come from milk-fed veal or young calves.

What people drink fresh blood?

If you watch the National Geographic Channel, you may already know about the Masai people of northern Tanzania, semi-nomadic herdsmen who keep cattle for use in trade and for their milk. It is rare that they would ever kill one of their highly prized animals, but they will nick a vein from time to time to drain a cup of blood, which is often mixed with the cow's own milk. Don't fret, this occasional blood-letting does the cow no harm. The fierce Mongol warriors of Genghis Khan also would occasionally partake in a cup of warm blood from one of their many horses while on a battle campaign.

Many modern cultures use blood as a main ingredient in a variety of soups and sausages. Polish blood soup, or *czarnina*, is one example. It's a soup containing duck's blood. Locals favor a pig's blood soup in Korea and the Philippines. Filipinos also enjoy a dish of congealed duck blood, served on a plate with lemon, herbs, and a rice cracker.

The Portuguese make a dish called *arroz de cabidela* (chicken with rice in blood). A chicken or duck is killed and its blood is collected in a container with a half a cup of vinegar. The meat is cut up and stewed with vegetables and rice. At the end of the cooking process, the blood is added. When the liquid starts to boil, the dish is removed from the heat.

Many cultures make blood sausage, in which the blood is cooked with a filler until it is thick enough to congeal when cooled. One such recipe is known as black pudding in England.

What is humble pie?

You may have had to swallow your pride from time to time, but it's probably better than eating real humble pie, which also has a little something to do with humility.

In jolly Old England, the landed gentry were quite found of deer meat. They would keep the venison for themselves and give the entrails, known as "umbles," to the lowly servants. It was common for the lower classes to make pie from these innards. It was called umble, or humble, pie because of their station in life.

Why do some cultures eat bugs?

Lots of cultures enjoy snacking on bugs. In Mexico, village markets sell grasshoppers by the pound. They are also sold fried in cans, as are caterpillars. Red and white agave worm tortillas can be found in Mexico City restaurants.

In the Philippines, ants, crickets, dragonfly larvae, grasshoppers, locusts, June beetles, katydids, and water beetles are all consumed. Similar bugs supplement diets in parts of Africa and Asia, as well.

Folks in Thailand enjoy rice bugs. These are large 4- to 6-inch insects that look like giant white cockroaches. They eat rice, hence their name. The Thai people don't actually eat the bug, but pop off its head and suck out the rice within.

Some Americans eat insects, but they all seem to be entomologists (who are a unique bunch, anyway). They will point out that insects are cleaner than other edible animals. Unlike lobsters, crabs, clams, and catfish, which scavenge all kinds of decomposing crud, grasshoppers and crickets eat only fresh, green grass.

Worldwide, about 1,462 different insect species are eaten. But not all bugs are edible. Some cause allergic reactions, while others are downright toxic. So if you're eager to start eating bugs, don't just run out into the backyard and fry up the first appetizing looking thing you see.

So, what are the benefits of eating bugs? The fancy

term for the eating of insects is *entomophagy*. Does that make them any easier to swallow? Then chew on this—insects have a higher food conversion efficiency than do other sources of protein. What the heck does that mean? Simply put, insects require less food of equal quality to produce the same weight of edible protein as compared to livestock. Insects also reproduce at a much faster rate than do livestock. A house cricket, for example, has a food conversion efficiency 20 times greater than that of a cow. Some caterpillars have the same amount of protein per pound as beef. Because insects are such an inexpensive source of protein, many cultures have incorporated them into their diets as a main dish or as a meat substitute. Plus they are low in cholesterol and fat!

Where do people eat fried ant bellies?

Colombians nosh on fried ant bellies at the movies, just like you might snack on Milk Duds. They also munch on termites, palm grubs, and ants that are ground up and spread on bread. Other South American culinary curiosities include tarantulas (see page 23) and their eggs, which are eaten by people in the Brazilian rain forest.

Feel like you are missing out on the culinary fun? One quick and easy (or "queasy") snack you can whip up some summer day is fried grasshoppers. They are much loved around the world. The hardest part may be catching them. Once you get a few, pull off their wings, head, small legs, and the lower part of their hind legs. Brown them lightly in a frying pan with some oil. To make them extra yummy, add a dash of salt. You could even sneak a bucketful into the movie theater next time you go and skip paying the 10 bucks for popcorn.

Who eats tarantulas?

There are almost 900 species of tarantula found around the world. Some cultures enjoy them as a delicacy. The Piaroa people of Venezuela fancy the goliath bird-eating tarantula (*Theraphosa leblondi*). Locals lure the spider out of its tunnel with a long blade of grass, then carefully pick it up by its thorax, bend the legs back, and wrap it up in a leaf for easy transport back to the campfire.

The eggs are cooked separately, wrapped in a leaf, to yield a tarantula egg omelet. The body is thrown on the coals to singe off the hair and roast the meat. When done, the spider is dismembered and eaten by picking out the bits of meat, like a crab. It tastes something like shrimp or crab. The long fangs make handy toothpicks.

In the Sukon region of eastern Thailand, street vendors sell hundreds of tarantulas a day. The eating of spiders is also very popular in neighboring Cambodia. During the terror reign of the Khmer Rouge in the late 1970s, food was very scarce and the people began foraging for the large spiders to supplement their diet. Since then, tarantulas have become a national delicacy. They are fried in butter with garlic, salt, and MSG and are sold by the basketful.

Crispy on the outside and gooey on the inside, spiders are a dish best served hot. There is little meat in the legs, but the body and head have a delicate white meat inside. The abdomen is more of an acquired taste. It contains a brown paste made up of the organs, eggs, and excrement. At a street price of 8 cents (U.S.) each, however, how can you go wrong?!

Can you eat stinkbugs?

Stinkbugs, if you don't already know, are beetle-like bugs that emit an obnoxious gas when crushed or handled roughly, thus earning their name. For this reason, most people don't squish them but gently gather them up and throw them outside or flush them down the toilet. Other people enjoy eating them.

If you ever find yourself in the Venda region of South Africa, you may want to try the local edible stinkbug dishes. Stinkbugs spend the winter in the adult stage and don't go underground like other insects. This means fully grown stinkbugs can be harvested in winter when little other food is available.

The women of Venda gather the stinkbugs by hand before dawn, when the critters are less active. The stinkbug's defensive secretions turn the women's hands orange. The live bugs are placed in a bucket with a small amount of warm water and stirred with a wooden spoon. This alarms the bugs and they release their noxious gases. The women can become overpowered by the secretions and must turn their heads away and close their eyes. The bugs are rinsed, and the process is repeated three times. Then the insects are boiled in water, which kills them, and dried in the sun.

The preparation is good only for live stinkbugs. Dead ones must be handled differently. The heads are removed, and the thorax and abdomen are squeezed until a pale green gland pops out of the neck of the dead insect. It is rubbed off on a rock. Then the bugs are boiled and sun dried as described.

Dried stinkbugs make handy snacks when munched as is. They can also be fried in a little salted water and served with pap, a traditional porridge made from *mielie meal* (cornmeal). Other African cultures use the bugs to add flavor to stews.

What people like to eat ticks and lice before sex?

Most people like to share food before sex. A nice romantic dinner maybe or breakfast in bed. But ticks and lice? Members of the Siriono tribe in eastern Bolivia groom each other, picking off bugs and eating them, before engaging in intercourse. This is the extent of their foreplay. They don't hug, kiss, or fondle. (Much like some married couples you may know.)

What is maggot cheese?

The food with the grossest name is maggot cheese, or *casu marzu*, as its devotees call it. Pecorino cheese is left out under cheesecloth so that cheese flies (*Piophila casei*) can lay their eggs in it. Once the maggots hatch, they help ferment the cheese and break down its fats, making it quite soft textured.

When sufficiently ripe, the cheese, including the live maggots, is spread on bread. The transparent-white maggots can jump up to 6 inches when disturbed, so some diners wear glasses to protect their eyes!

Who would eat anything this disgusting? Folks in Sardinia, that's who.

How many insect parts do you inadvertently eat?

Humans have been supplementing their diet with insects since time immemorial. In our scavenging past, before we settled down and began farming, insects would have been one of the easiest forms of food protein around. Coprolites (that's scientific jargon for fossilized doo-doo) show that our ancestors used to regularly eat things like ants, beetle larvae, lice, mites, and ticks. Although some cultures still enjoy such fare, Westerners consider themselves "above" such primitive vittles. Alas, this disdain for insects notwithstanding, Westerners still inadvertently eat plenty of insect material every year.

Loads of insect parts, and lots of other gross stuff, finds its way into your food. Most of it is allowed by law. The U.S. Food and Drug Administration (FDA) has set standards for the allowable amounts of insect parts or rodent filth permitted in your food. Called the Food Defect Action Level, these are the tolerance levels allowed before an FDA investigation will begin to examine for a problem.[5] The following is a sampling of what the government has decided it's OK for you to ingest before they start investigating:

- *Chocolate:* 60 or more insect fragments per 100 grams; 1 or more rodent hairs per 100 grams
- *Citrus juices:* 5 or more fly eggs, or 1 or more maggots, per 250 milliliters
- *Broccoli (frozen):* average of 60 or more aphids and/ or thrips and/or mites per 100 grams
- *Popcorn:* 1 or more rodent excreta pellets in 1 or more subsamples and 1 or more rodent hairs in 2 or more other subsamples, or 2 or more rodent hairs per pound and rodent hair in 50 percent or more of subsamples, or 20 or more gnawed grains per pound and rodent hair in 50 percent or more of the subsamples—Got all that? Well, you can just draw the conclusion that there may be plenty of rodents droppings, hair, and gnawed kernels in your mouth next time you munch on that $10 tub o' popcorn at your local cinema.

Think those numbers sound pretty low? Here's some food for thought—a University of Ohio study found that each of us unwittingly consumes between 1 and 2 pounds of insects each year.[6] Eating these insect parts may cause some of you to have allergic reactions or upset stomachs. Thinking about it may have the same effect.

Where do they sell octopus ice cream?

If you guessed Japan, give yourself two points. The Japanese have available to them a wide variety of crazy ice cream flavors. In addition to octopus, they can buy cactus, chicken wing, corn, crab, eel, fish, fried eggplant, ox tongue, shrimp, squid, and wasabi ice creams. Almost makes you want to jump on the next plane to the Far East!

What people enjoy live octopus?

If you guessed the South Koreans, give yourself another two points. They enjoy a dish called *sannakji*. It is prepared by cutting up a small live octopus and serving it with sesame oil, while the tentacles are still wiggling. One note of caution: If you are contemplating whipping up some *sannakji* for the family, be aware that the tentacle's suction cups still function and may stick to the inside of your mouth or the back or your throat. There is a definite choking hazard, particularly if you have been drinking to excess, which may be the only way to stomach this dish. *Bon appétit!*

Who eats live shrimp?

One of the reasons so many Chinese dishes seem off-the-charts bizarre to Westerners is because they're not used to them. One such dish is drunken shrimp.

The name is apt. You'd have to be pretty darn drunk not to feel a bit squeamish when eating this creepy dish. It's served in Shanghai-style restaurants and really does consist of drunken shrimp. Not only are the shrimp served raw but they are still alive! If you order drunken shrimp, they will arrive at your table swimming in a bowl of sweet alcohol. (Not a bad way to go if you have to be eaten alive.) The booze not only adds flavoring to the crustaceans but makes them a little less feisty when you try to eat them. They should remain in their alcohol bath for at least 5 minutes before eating.

Even in their inebriated state, the shrimp still put up a fight and will pinch the careless diner. They are removed from the bowl with chopsticks and plated. You should remove the head with your fingers before popping the still twitching body into your mouth. Nothing like live meat to sate the carnivorous appetite.

Why do Native Alaskans suffer from the highest rate of botulism in the world?

Stink heads. Sounds like some new gross kid's candy. In reality, stink heads are fermented salmon heads, a traditional Inuit food from southwestern Alaska.

Along with stink heads, the locals also enjoy other fermented morsels, such as stink eggs (fish eggs), stinky tail (beaver tail), *muktuk* (whale blubber), and seal flipper. Animals are often slaughtered on the beach or on the ground, where the meat comes in contact with bacteria from the sand or soil. The food is then placed in a cool, shallow pit in the ground, lined with wood, animal skin, or leaves. It is covered with moss and left to "ferment" for a month or two. The foods don't really ferment; the process of fermentation requires sugars, which these foods don't possess. What they actually do is just rot in the ground.

Traditionally, this fermentation served the purpose of providing essential nutrients missing from the native diet. Fermented fish heads have softened bones that can be eaten for a good source of calcium. The process may also release some vitamin B. However, stink head fermentation offers the perfect conditions for the growth of *Clostridium,* the bacterium responsible for botulism, which is anaerobic, meaning it thrives in an oxygen-free environment.

Ironically, modern Native Alaskans are using plastic

to line their holes or simply placing the foods in jars to speed up the decomposition process. This provides an even more oxygen-free environment for the bacteria in which to flourish. Consequently, the rate of botulism in Alaska increased by 12 times between 1966 and 1988, according to a 1988 report in the *Journal of Infectious Diseases*.[7]

Botulism is nothing new in Alaska. Early explorers noted entire families that were wiped out by what is now presumed to have been botulism. Botulism affects nerve transmission, causing weakness, paralysis, and sometimes death. Symptoms appear within 18 to 36 hours of ingesting the toxin, which binds to nerve endings and blocks impulses from one nerve to the next. The first symptoms may be nausea, vomiting, abdominal cramps, and diarrhea, followed by drooping eyelids, difficulty in swallowing, dry mouth, vertigo, dizziness, and lassitude. It then moves downward, and the limbs become paralyzed, followed by the muscles of the chest and diaphragm. Respiratory failure and pneumonia are the greatest threats to life.

Unfortunately, efforts to get Native Alaskans to change their traditions have met with resistance. They feel that outsiders are trying to interfere with their culture. So disease rates remain high.

What people love cod tongues?

Canadians, that's who. Well, not all Canadians. Cod tongues are a localized dish popular on the island of

Newfoundland. The dish is quite simple to prepare. Just get a bunch of cod tongues (you'll have to cut them out of cod heads); wash them; coat with flour, salt, and pepper; and fry up in a pan with salt pork. Plan on 6 to 8 tongues per person.

Because you have got a bunch of tongueless cod heads lying around anyway, why not whip up some cod cheeks while you're at it? They're also a snap to prepare. Yep, cods have cheeks, and you'll have to remove them. For this recipe, you roll the cheeks in a mixture of eggs, cream, mustard, dill, and basil and fry them in butter. Both dishes are served with potatoes and peas.

Now you've got a meal that's a little tongue in cheek.

What soup is made from birds' nests?

There's one Asian delicacy that is quite unique. It's called bird's nest soup, and it really is made from the nest of a bird. It has been a traditional Chinese dish for over 1,000 years. Aficionados believe the soup has restorative properties and raises libido.

The cave swiftlet, or swift, is a little Asian bird that builds its nest on the sides of cave walls. The male bird builds the nest. Unlike the traditional stick-and-mud bird's nest you may be accustomed to (and which wouldn't be edible) the cave swift constructs a nest made of its gummy saliva, which hardens when exposed to air. It takes the male 35 days to build the small half-cup-shaped nest. There are two types of nests—black and white. The black nests are built by the black-nest swiftlet (*Aerodramus maxima*) and the white nests by the edible-nest swiftlet (*Aerodramus fushipagus*). The white nests are more desirable because the black nests are full of feathers that must be removed.

These nests are not easy to come by. Harvesting them is very difficult and dangerous. Some of them are built over 100 feet up the walls of dark caverns. This scarcity and the difficulty in collecting have made the nests one of the most expensive foods in the world. In Hong Kong, a bowl of bird's nest soup will run you from $30 to $100.

Dissolved in water, the nests have a gelatinous texture. Because they don't have much taste, the nests are often simmered in chicken broth and spices. They have little nutritional value.

Can you get a disease from a fly in your soup?

There are about as many punch lines to the old joke, "Waiter, there's a fly in my soup!" as there are diseases you can contract *from* a fly in your soup. As you all know, flies get around. They are as much attracted to a fresh steaming pile of manure as they are to your peanut butter and jelly sandwich.

Flies taste with their feet. (Their sense of taste is said to be 10,000 times more sensitive than our own.) This is why flies walk around on stuff so much—they are tasting it. Because flies don't have teeth, biting mouth parts, or sucking tubes, they must live on a liquid diet.

When a fly finds something it likes, it vomits up some of its stomach's digestive juices and uses its sponge-like tongue to lap up the dissolved food. The only problem is, the fly may have been tasting and lapping up rotting garbage or dog poop just before walking around and barfing on your hamburger. When it pukes up digestive juices, it also spits out some of the leftover food from its last meal, which could have been almost any disgusting thing you care to think of.

Flies are able to walk on the ceiling because their hairy legs and feet ooze a sticky, slimy substance. These hairy legs and gooey feet trap a lot of germs from the surfaces the fly walks on, meaning they also spread these same germs from one place to the next.

Researchers had houseflies scamper around on a sterile Petri dish filled with agar. In a few days' time, they could see trails of bacteria where the flies had walked. In fact, it has been shown that the average housefly has about 1.25 million bacteria on its body.

If you consider all this at your next outdoor picnic, ants may be the least of your worries. Place a paper napkin over your plate to keep the flies off your food. If one of these germ couriers does alight on your potato salad, you'd be wise to remove that little bit and throw it away.

Do they really grow mushrooms in manure?

You bet! We may not love manure, but mushrooms sure do. So instead of raising them in topsoil, commercial growers mix together old farm debris—things like corncobs, hay, chicken droppings, and, yes, manure from the stables. Sounds appetizing, no? Well don't fret. It's all perfectly safe. Mushroom growth medium is composted for a few weeks and then pasteurized before the fungal spores are sewn, killing any dangerous microorganisms.

Now, you've all seen that brown dirt-like stuff that's on fresh store-bought mushrooms. And you've probably wondered if it is manure. Remain calm. This is just peat moss that the growers spread over the mushroom beds to keep them moist. The mushroom caps grow through the moss before they are picked. A quick rinse is all that's needed.

FYI: Mushrooms are grown indoors, in the dark. Half of the country's mushroom crop comes from Pennsylvania: Kennett Square is billed as the Mushroom Capital of the World.

What fruit's original name means "testicle"?

Think guacamole. Yes, it's the avocado (*Persea americana*). It is a member of the laurel family that is native to Central America. The Aztecs enjoyed eating avocados and called them *ahuacatl,* their word for "testicle," which they somewhat resemble. The Spaniards twisted the word into *aguacate.* This evolved into the present-day *avocado,* certainly a more appetizing name than the original.

What's the deal with those green potato chips?

Opening a bag of fresh, golden, crunchy potato chips is one of life's simple pleasures. Once in a while though, you'll pull out one of those "mutant" green chips. If you are normal, you will make a face and toss it back in the bag for some other unsuspecting snacker. But did you ever wonder where these alien chips come from?

Potatoes, as you know, grow in the dark, under the soil. Sometimes, however, a bit of the tuber will stick up above the soil line and be exposed to sunlight. This causes that part of the potato to produce chlorophyll and turn green. Chlorophyll isn't bad for you, but the chemical solanine that is produced in these green spots isn't that great for you in large quantities. There are no definitive studies on how many green chips it would take to make you sick, but why not play it safe and throw it back in the bag anyway?

Those dark brown chips also pop up once in a while. They are quite harmless. These result when a potato has been in storage too long and starts to build up sugars. The high sugar content makes the chips turn dark brown when cooked.

What popular kid's dessert is made from bones and hooves?

Gelatin is made from cow and pig hooves and bones. Yum! Gelatin, like glue, is made by boiling the bones, hooves, connective tissue, and hides in strong acids and bases to release the protein-rich collagen from their tissues. After repeated boiling and filtering, the collagen is partially broken down into gelatin, which is dried and powdered.

Collagen is a big, fibrous molecule that gives bones, tendons, and skin their elasticity. You might be aware of collagen, or the lack or it, as you age and your skin becomes less elastic—that is, wrinkled.

Gelatin is a most versatile ingredient in foods. It can be used as a gelling agent, as an emulsifier, as a stabilizer, and as a thickener. It is found in candies, meats, dairy products, sauces, gravies, frostings, cosmetics, and even the clear coating on pills that makes them easy to swallow.

The FDA doesn't consider gelatin to be an animal product because it has been processed so extensively, but many ardent vegetarians avoid it in all its many incarnations.

What dish is made from the heads of calves and pigs?

There's no cheese in headcheese, but there *is* a lot of head. It's actually a sausage made from the meaty bits of pig or calf heads (sometimes sheep or cow).

The head meat and skull have a lot of cartilage, ligaments, and muscle that turns into a clear, gelatinous substance when cooked. Chilling it makes it harden into a kind of meat gelatin.

Modern headcheese is made from the meats of the head, minus the brains, and edible parts of the hoof, tongue, and heart. They are cooked with a gelatin and molded into a lunch-meat product. Headcheese can be purchased in supermarkets. It is usually sliced thin and eaten at room temperature on a sandwich. It is popular in England and among the Pennsylvania Dutch.

Where is there a restaurant that serves nothing but genitals?

The eating of animal genitalia goes back at least to ancient Rome, when it was believed that eating an animal's member would help improve an ailment in the diner's own. This belief is alive and well in Asia, particularly in China. According to *China Daily*, Guo-li-zhuang's, in Beijing, is China's first specialty penis restaurant.[8] You want penis? They got penis. In fact, every dish on the menu has some kind of penis or testicle in it. They got yak and oxen dick, horse and donkey schlong, even dog and seal dong.

In China, you are what you eat. Clients are mainly men who wish to improve their yang, or virility. Diners get a nutritionist who explains the medicinal virtues of each dish. For first-timers, they recommend their sample platter: the hot pot, which consists of a variety of six penises and four testicles in chicken broth.

Why do some people eat dirt?

When you think of eating dirt, you probably think of young kids. Although some of them do indeed eat dirt, many adults in Central Africa, India, Turkey, and the rural American South also engage in the eating of dirt, or *geophagy*, as it is properly known.

You may be familiar with the strange cravings of pregnant women. Well, in Africa, pregnant and breast-feeding women eat clay to satisfy their body's needs for additional nutrients. They also eat it to ease morning sickness. It works by buffering the gastrointestinal tract and absorbing toxins. The dirt comes from favored clay pits, is labeled with its nutrient content, and is sold in markets. Women keep their clay in special belt-like cloths worn around their waists. This way they can nibble on dry clay throughout the day. These African clays contain such nutrients as copper, iron, magnesium, manganese, phosphorus, potassium, and zinc. Some clays also contain calcium, which is not found in the diets of many sub-Saharan tribes.

These are not the only people who eat dirt. Some Native Americans, like the Pomo of northern California, used dirt when making acorn bread to neutralize the seed's natural tannin acid content. The Andean peoples of South America use dirt when preparing potatoes to absorb the toxic glycoalkaloid solanine found in their native potatoes.

Unfortunately, some people eat dirt because they suffer from pica, an eating disorder in which they're compelled to eat soil and non-nutritive things, like laundry starch, chalk, ashes, cigarette butts, burned match heads, and paint chips, which have no nutritional value and can lead to intestinal difficulties or lead poisoning.

Did you ever eat dirt?

If you ever used Kaopectate you did. Clay was an active ingredient in some antidiarrheal medicines. Kaopectate used to be made from kaolin (attapulgite clay) and pectin, hence the name. Very recently, pink bismuth subsalicylate (the stuff in Pepto-Bismol) has replaced the clay, which was found to contain unsafe levels of lead.

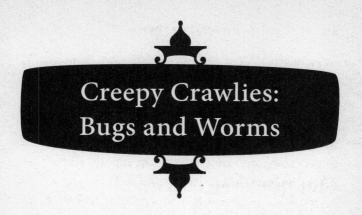

Creepy Crawlies: Bugs and Worms

Some bugs, such as butterflies and fireflies, are a source of beauty and awe. They are innocuous and rarely interact with us, save when we stop to admire them. Other insects are more nefarious and are intimately involved in our lives. These parasites, along with many worms, make a living feeding on us. Almost every major culture abhors these creepy crawlies. Whether you realize it or not, you are rife with millions of tiny vermin that are—right at this very moment—walking, crawling, breeding, feeding, and excreting all over (and within) you. If you tend to get itchy easily, prepare to start scratching.

What creatures come out of your anus at night?

There is a parasite that lives in your lower small intestine and upper colon; and like many other creepy creatures, it comes out only at night.

You've most likely heard of pinworms, also known as threadworms (genus *Enterobius*). They are most commonly found in children, who spread them to each other through eggs picked up under the fingernails while playing. The eggs are then ingested when the fingers come into contact with the mouth, where they hatch and start the infection process.

The male pinworm is 1 to 4 millimeters long; the female, 8 to 13 millimeters. After mating, the male dies and the female wiggles her way out during the night and lays between 10,000 and 20,000 eggs around your anus! Over these she secretes a chemical that causes profound itching.

The itching has an evolutionary purpose. When you scratch the itch in your sleep, you will unwittingly get some of the eggs under your fingernails. Odds are your fingers will eventually make it to your mouth, thus causing reinfection. Once ingested, these little worms hatch and migrate down your throat and esophagus to the intestines and mature in 30 to 45 days, beginning the pinworm's life cycle all over again. Pinworm eggs can remain viable for 2 to 3 weeks under your nails, on your sheets and clothes, and in the bathtub. Sometimes, the eggs around your anus will hatch right there and the worms will wiggle their way back up your rectum (!) and into the intestines to mature. Young girls face the added risk of an adult worm wiggling its way into her vagina, instead of her rectum, causing irritation and discomfort.

If all this information weren't gross enough for you, how about this? If you want to check for pinworms, try the "Scotch tape test." Wake up from sleep some night and press a piece of cellophane tape against your perianal area (butt hole). The eggs will adhere and can be seen under a microscope. Ask your doctor, if you wish to see them. To check for pinworms on your kids, wait till they have been asleep a couple of hours, then shine a flashlight between their cheeks (at their rectums) and look for a whitish material that moves. (Yikes!)

Pinworms are the most common worm infection in North America and Europe. It is estimated that over 40 million Americans, mostly children, are infected annually. The problem is so ubiquitous that there are several over-the-counter medications available.

So what's the moral of this story? Don't scratch your ass in your sleep and thoroughly wash your hands often, especially upon awakening!

What worm lives in your intestines and may crawl out of your nose?

The *Ascaris lumbricoides* roundworm affects up to one-quarter of the world's population every year. It is especially prevalent in tropical regions and poor areas where hygiene is lacking. It has been estimated that roughly 4 million Americans are infected, mainly in the Ozark Mountains and Gulf Coast regions.

These little devils cause a disease known as ascariasis. They enter the body when you ingest their eggs in fecal material. Once in your belly, they hatch; tunnel through your intestinal wall; make their way to the liver, heart, and lungs; and then find their way into the respiratory tract. Now comes the disgusting part. They crawl up the back of your throat, giving you a tickling sensation that causes you to swallow them back down into your intestines. There they mature and latch on to your intestinal wall. These worms can grow to up to a foot long. If the tickle in the back of your throat causes you to cough instead of swallow, you make hack them up into your mouth! They are also expelled when you vomit.

Now for the really gross part. In heavy infestations, or if provoked by anesthesia or certain medications, the worms will flee the body through the mouth, nose, or even the corner of your eye! If they enter the trachea, they can cause suffocation. So, the next time you have a little tickle in your throat . . . you never know. (Do you feel a sudden urge to clear your throat? Thought so.)

Once mature, the females will lay from 200,000 to 2 million eggs a day, which you will pass in your feces. The egg-laden feces will contaminate the soil and water that it comes in contact with. The most common sources of infection are ingesting contaminated water, food, or soil. This is a great reason not to eat that piece of toast you drop on the floor, regardless of whether the buttered side lands up, or not. It's also a good reason to wash all produce that comes from any country in which soil and water may not be quite up to snuff.

What other parasite crawls into the back of your throat?

Are you fond of sashimi? More and more Westerners are these days. Properly handled, raw fish is safe. Proper handling, however, does not always occur, and improper preparation can have disgusting consequences. The U.S. Food and Drug Administration (FDA) recommends that all fish and shellfish intended for raw consumption be blast frozen to −31°F or below for at least 15 hours or be normally frozen at −4°F for at least 7 days.

What sense does it make to freeze fish that is supposed to be eaten fresh? The answer is the herring worm (*Anisakis simplex*) and cod worm (*Phocanema decipiens*). These guys are large, 2-centimeter-long (about an inch) roundworms that cause something called anisakiasis when humans ingest them.

The infestation is usually diagnosed when an affected person feels a tickling sensation in the back of his or her throat, which occurs when the nematodes (small worms) come crawling up. Folks who experience such a feeling, will either cough up the little buggers into their mouth or reach into the throat and manually extract them. In more severe cases, people can get acute abdominal pain, nausea, and vomiting within an hour or two of consumption. This is good because vomiting usually dislodges the worms. If, however, they manage to get into your bowel, you will develop severe gastrointestinal problems in 1 to 2 weeks' time. Worms that enter your bowel will stay there about 3 weeks. The only treatment is to physically remove them or just wait for them to die. One 58-year-old Japanese woman had 56 *Anisakis simplex* worms surgically removed from her stomach in 1990. She got them from sashimi.

Some people are highly allergic to these worms and can go into anaphylactic shock.

There are only about 10 documented cases of anisakiasis a year in the United States, but it is believed that numerous cases go undiagnosed or are misdiagnosed. The prevalence is much higher in Japan, where folks really love their raw seafood. (Maybe they should stick to blackened sea bass.)

What worms will form cysts in your muscles?

Did your mom ever freak out if your pork chop wasn't thoroughly cooked? This is because back in the old days, undercooked pork could give you something called trichinosis. It is about as bad as its name sounds.

Trichinosis is quite rare today; only about a dozen cases a year are reported in the United States. It is caused by eating meat that is infected with larvae of the *Trichinella* worm. These guys commonly occur in wild game and domestic pigs that have been fed raw meat garbage, a common practice years ago before it was outlawed.

The first symptoms of trichinosis, also called trichinellosis, include diarrhea, nausea, vomiting, fever, and fatigue and will be evident in 24 to 48 hours after infection. Subsequent symptoms—diarrhea or constipation, chills, fever, headaches, eye swelling, itchy skin, achy joints, muscle pain—follow in 2 to 8 weeks. (This infection has it all!) Severity of symptoms depends on the amount of worms consumed. Mild cases may be undiagnosed and put down as the flu.

Trichinella cysts live in the meat of infected animals. When you eat meat that contains active cysts, the acid in your stomach dissolves the cyst walls, releasing the worms. They pass into the small intestine and mature in a couple of days. After mating and egg laying, the worms find their way into your arteries, and from there, into your muscles, where they encyst.

Pork today is pretty safe, although you should still cook it until the juices run clear—about 170°F. It's wild meat you have to be more careful with. If bear, cougar, dog, fox, horse, seal, walrus, or wolf meat is on your menu, beware—they are all sources of infection.

What worm can grow to 50 feet long inside you?

A tapeworm is a segmented, flat, ribbon-like worm. Hence the name. Its eggs and larvae can be ingested in contaminated water, undercooked meats and fish, or soil contaminated with feces. Once in the body, a tapeworm migrates to your intestines, where it attaches its head by means of hooks and/or suckers. Tapeworms can be up to 50 feet long and live for 20 years!

Most infestations are asymptomatic, but sometimes diarrhea, nausea, and abdominal cramps can occur.

Tapeworms from beef (*Taenia saginata*) usually do not cause many problems, but pork tapeworms (*Taenia solium*) may cause complications.

If you think you may have a tapeworm, look at your stool (that's medicalese for poop). You may see eggs, larvae, or body segments. (Eew!) Better yet, see a doctor. There are medicines available to quickly rid your body of these beasties.

Jewish women used to get something called "Jewish housewife's disease." Because they frequently tasted raw gefilte fish before cooking it, they became infested with the freshwater fish tapeworm *Diphyllobothrium latum*.

What is a tapeworm diet?

There were rumors in the 1950s that certain celebrities were losing weight by taking a tapeworm pill. Would that really work? Yes, you would lose weight, but at what cost? Not only will a tapeworm take in some of the food you eat but it will also rob you of some vitamins and minerals. Worse than this, a tapeworm in your gut will cause an immune response from your body that will result in a pool of fluid, giving you a big potbelly. Worse still, a tapeworm can cause cysts in your liver, muscles, and eyes. Muscle cysts can form bumps under the skin. Cysts in the eyes can float into your field of vision.

Legend has it that opera star Maria Callas (1923–1977) lost 65 pounds by taking a tapeworm pill. Historians believe she may have accidentally ingested a tapeworm in the raw steak and liver that she was fond of eating. After Callas lost all that weight, she dumped her husband and began an affair with the then-married shipping tycoon Aristotle Onassis. He in turn dumped her for former First Lady Jackie Kennedy. (But we digress.)

What condition can swell a man's testicles to 2 feet in diameter?

If the thought of a tapeworm in your gut grosses you out, elephantitis will make your head spin. Perhaps you have heard of this *most* bizarre condition. It, too, is the result of worms, specifically *Wuchereria bancrofti, Brugia malayi,* and *Brugia timori.* Worldwide, some 120 million people are infected and 40 million seriously so.

These little buggers are transmitted in the tropics via mosquito bites. A female mosquito injects the worm larvae into your bloodstream, where they begin to reproduce. There may be no symptoms for years. Eventually, there will be so many of these little guys in your blood vessels that they will restrict circulation and cause the buildup of fluids, particularly in the arms, legs, breasts, and genitals.

Infected tissues may become enlarged to the extreme. Cases of testicles swollen to 2 feet in diameter and weighing over 150 pounds are documented! There are numerous websites to visit if you wish to see some horrific pictures of this condition. (Just type *elephantitis* into

your browser's search engine.) Drugs to treat elephantitis are effective if used early, but most cases are too far
advanced for treatment before detection.

What human parasite causes you to want to eat dirt?

Hookworms are ½-inch-long worms called nematodes.
They make their living in your small intestine. There
are two species of hookworms that may attack you:
Ancylostoma duodenale and *Necator americanus*. They
are prevalent in sandy, loamy tropical soils.

Most people who have hookworm infestations aren't
even aware of it. Unless you have a high level of infestation, you will be asymptomatic. Those with symptoms
will experience pain in the stomach, constipation followed by diarrhea, palpitations, anemia, and something called pica—a strange desire to eat dirt, which is
especially common in children. This craving may be in
response to the iron deficiency created by the worms
sucking blood out of the gut.

Hookworms affect about 1 billion people worldwide. They cause premature and underweight births
in infected mothers and intellectual, cognitive, and
growth retardation in infected children. Heavily
infected children will often develop a potbelly and an
emaciated body.

Hookworms are spread through eggs in human feces.
The eggs hatch in the stool, and larvae enter the soil,
where they wait for you to step on them with bare feet or

otherwise touch soil containing them. They then penetrate your skin, get into your bloodstream, and head for your heart and then your lungs. From the lungs they make their way into your pharynx, where you swallow them. Next, they move from your stomach into your small intestine, where they latch onto the walls of your intestine and suck the blood out of you for several years. Adults lay eggs that pass out of you in your excrement to infect more unsuspecting souls/soles.

Why do some people intentionally drink intestinal worms?

Studies in Ethiopia have found that people affected with hookworms are much less likely to suffer from asthma.[1] It seems that our immune systems evolved under stress from a variety of parasites. These parasites also evolved to live in us by causing our immune systems to slow down. In the modern world, we are not as exposed to the many parasites our ancestors were: Kids used to always run around barefoot and drink from a spring or a stream. Now our water and food is very clean and we have fewer parasites. When the parasites are not present or are removed, our immune systems are not suppressed and may begin to attack our own tissues, resulting in problems like asthma, hay fever, colitis, Crohn's disease, and possibly other autoimmune diseases. In other words, this theory says that some parasites are really good for us and keep our immune systems in check, or at least in a proper balance.

Ulcerative colitis is a disease of the intestine caused by the immune system working overtime. The white blood cells attack the gut as if it were a foreign invader, causing it to bleed. The disease is incurable, but researchers have come up with a novel, if a bit disgusting, treatment.

Volunteers in a University of Iowa study found that by downing a drink of 2,500 pig whipworm eggs, every 3 weeks for 24 weeks, symptoms could be lessened.[2] The worms, which are harmless intestinal parasites, grow in the gut and seem to make the immune system kick down a notch or two, providing relief to colitis suffers. Bottoms up!

What bugs burrow under your skin and cause unbelievable itching?

Scabies: Just the name sounds gross, and you'd better believe it is. The word *scabies* is Greek for "itch." It may be the itchiest condition known to man (and woman).

Scabies is a skin disorder caused by wingless bugs called human itch mites or scabies itch mites—*Sarcoptes scabiei* var. *hominis*. What happens when you get scabies? The female mite burrows under your skin and lays one to three eggs a day for 5 weeks. A very small, zigzag blister marks the trail of the mite as she tunnels along laying her eggs. It is usually very hard to see with the naked eye. The eggs hatch in 3 to 10 days and start the cycle all over again. The male mites just roam around on the surface of your skin cruising for females, although they, too, sometimes like to burrow. The females will surface at night and hook up with the males.

You will have no symptoms of scabies for 4 to 6 weeks after infection. Then you will experience unbelievable itching. The motion of the mites on your skin and a massive allergic reaction to the presence of the eggs under your skin produce the intense itch.

Scabies most frequently occurs on the wrists, ankles, elbows, armpits, waistline, inner thighs, between the fingers, on the backs of the hands, around the areolae of the nipples in women, and on the genitals in men. (Yikes!)

Scabies is spread by prolonged skin-to-skin contact. You will not get it from just shaking someone's hand. It is generally spread to sexual partners or family members. In some instances, it can be transmitted through shared clothing, bedding, combs, brushes, and so on. This usually is not the case, however, because the mites can't live for long off of a human host.

If you think you may have scabies, see your doctor because it is difficult to diagnose at home. The mites and their eggs are very small. The doctor will have to put mineral oil on one of the blisters and scrape off the skin below. The scrapings are then put on a slide and examined under a microscope, as the zigzag blister trails can't often be found with the naked eye. Then your doctor will rub a blue or black felt-tipped pen over the suspected area. Upon cleaning, the mite burrows are revealed if the ink sinks into them.

Scabies is treated with topical pesticide ointments that must be applied to the entire body from head to toe, or with oral medications. Thorough washing of bedding, brushes, combs, and the like is also necessary to prevent reinfection.

Many people think that they can get scabies from their dog, and they're right! Humans can't get many infections from their dogs, but scabies is one notable exception. Dogs get a form of scabies called mange. Dog scabies mites will indeed burrow under your skin if given the chance. They cannot, however, live for long on a human host. After several days, they will die off, but not without causing you to itch for a couple of weeks.

How many dust mites are there in your pillow?

Caution: This entry is likely to make your skin crawl if you are squeamish. Even you more hardy folks may run out and buy a new pillow after reading this one. You have been warned!

Mites are arachnids, in the same family of bugs as ticks and spiders. Arachnids are not insects. All arachnids have eight legs, whereas insects have only six.

House dust mites are microscopic bugs that are 0.01 inch in length. You might just be able to see one with a 10 magnifying glass, if the mite were on a well-lit, black background. Under a microscope, you will see these oval-shaped creatures scurrying over and around each other, with their eight hairy legs and tough translucent shells. They are creamy white and globular in shape.

Dust mites live on the dead skin cells you constantly shed. (The average person sheds 50,000 skin flakes every minute, or 1.5 grams a day. Between 80 and 90 percent of the stuff you see floating in a sunbeam is dead skin flakes.) Mites inhabit the areas where your skin cells and scales, known as dander, accumulate—your pillow, mattress, sofa, carpeting, and the like.

Close to 100,000 dust mites can reside in 1 square yard of carpeting. The typical mattress may have anywhere from 100,000 to 10 million of these creepy crawlies inside. (Getting itchy yet?) That's nothing—10 percent of the weight of a 2-year-old pillow may be composed of dead mites and their feces! (Now you can start scratching.) They love pillows because your perspiration and hot breath give them plenty of the moisture they need to breed. While quite gross to think about, they actually do you a service by getting rid of much of your sloughed off skin that would otherwise create even more house dust.

Each of these tiny scavengers deposits 20 or more fecal droppings a day, which contain a protein to which many people are allergic. Symptoms range from itchy eyes to asthma attacks.

Take heart. House mites don't actually harm most people. They are a major component of house dust. Other constituents of house dust that may cause allergic reactions are cat dander, cockroach droppings, and pollen. Symptoms of house dust allergies are mainly respiratory in nature—sneezing, wheezing, itching and watery eyes, nasal congestion, and cough. The wheeze-inducing allergens come from the digestive juices of the mite. Exposure to mites during the first year of life can result in a life-long allergy problem for which there is no cure.

There are fewer house mites in arid climates than in humid ones. Likewise, their numbers go down in the drier months of winter. They will supplement their diet of dead skin cells with fungi, dog food, cereal, and other crumbs.

Just so you know, Americans are covered in different dust mites than are Europeans. The North American house dust mite is *Dermatophagoides farinae* and the European house dust mite is *Dermatophagoides pteronyssinus*. The genus name literally means "skin-eating"—from the Greek *derma,* meaning "layer of skin," and *phagos,* meaning "to eat."

The most effective way to protect yourself from house mites is to put a physical barrier between you and them. Enclosing your pillow, mattress, and furniture in plastic or polyurethane is one option (if you don't mind your living room looking like Marie Barone's). Specially made covers are available online. Washing your pillows and other bedding once a week in very hot water will also help. Bleach and strong soaps do not kill them. Sunlight does. You can also use a dehumidifier in your house. More drastic steps include replacing your carpeting with hard flooring or steam cleaning your carpets and drapes often. Freezing kills mites, so putting your pillow or child's stuffed toys in the freezer for a while couldn't hurt. Good luck.

Are there mites in your eyebrows?

If the thought of little bugs cavorting in your pillow creeped you out, you'll love reading about eyebrow mites. Around 98 percent of adults have these little creatures. These guys are real specialists, living primarily in the hair follicles and the adjacent sebaceous glands of the eyebrows, eyelashes, and around the nose. They are called *Demodex* mites. About 0.3 millimeters long, with stumpy little legs, claws, and needle-like mouth parts, their bodies are covered with scales the bugs use to anchor themselves to a host. *Demodex folliculorum* are found in hair follicles and *Demodex brevis* are found in the connected sebaceous glands. There, they use their mouths to puncture epithelial cells and suck up the fluids. Their digestive system is so efficient that the mites don't generate any waste at all, meaning they have no need for an excretory opening. (That's a plus.) They also lay their eggs on you and live out their short lives, their dead bodies left to decompose inside your hair follicles or sebaceous glands.

So how do these facial specialists spread from person to person? The easiest way is face-to-face contact—nuzzling. Because these mites are also found around the nipples, newborns can get a little more from mom than just milk. Once a mite finds itself on a new face, it immediately heads for the nearest hair follicle and dives in, so to speak.

Eyebrow mites are much more likely to be found on older people because children do not produce as much sebum as do adults. If you'd like to see your eyebrow mites, all you need is a microscope. Simply pluck out an eyebrow hair, or eyelash, pop it on a slide, and behold the horror.

What are lice?

A lot of kids think the opposite sex has "cooties." Actually, many of them do. (See why on page 61.) *Cootie* is another name for the blood-sucking head louse (*Pediculus humanus capitis*). It acquired this nickname from the British navy during World War I. The word *lousy* originally meant "louse-filled."

If the thought of little bugs living in your hair and sucking your blood disgusts you, read on. The head louse is a tiny (between 1 and 2 millimeters long—less than 0.1 inch), flat, wingless parasite that inhabits human hair and scalps. Lice are far more common than you may think on children between the ages of 3 and 12 years. They do not spread disease but are highly contagious little suckers. Their bites may cause redness and itching on the scalp but no serious problems.

So how do you know if you have lice? Well, you may feel things moving around on, or tickling, your head. Although very small, lice can be seen with the naked eye. Lice eggs, called "nits," are laid by adults on the hair shaft, close to the scalp. They are very small and look like tan or brown dots. Nymphs hatch from the eggs in 1 to 2 weeks and begin sucking blood from the scalp every 4 to 6 hours. Lice feed by sticking one straw-like mouth part into the scalp and injecting an anti-coagulant to keep the blood flowing, and another that they stick into a blood vessel to suck with.

To spot lice, spread the hair apart and shine a bright light on the scalp. Look behind the ears and around the nape of the neck. They are fast for their size and may scamper out of sight before you can see them.

Treatment involves medicated shampoos and fine combs to physically remove the lice and their eggs. If someone becomes infested, shaving the head bald is an option. They don't live long off the body, so you shouldn't need to fumigate the house or anything else.

How does one acquire head lice? Girls are more prone to lice infestations than boys. This is because girls are more likely to play dress-up, do each other's hair, and share clothing. It only takes one infested child at a sleepover; the rest of kids are easy targets. Some people think cats and dogs spread lice, but this is not the case. Head lice don't care for animal hair.

Are bedbugs making a comeback?

"Sleep tight, don't let the bedbugs bite." This old say-ing is about as close as many of us have gotten to a bed-bug. But, unfortunately, they are still around. Bedbugs came over to North America with the colonists, but were largely eradicated in the United States after World War II, with the extensive use of the pesticide DDT. Other areas of the globe have not been so fortunate. The recent increase in international travel and less-effective pesticides have contributed to a resurgence of bedbugs. They are most prevalent in dwellings with a high rate of turnover, like hotels, dormitories, and prisons.

The common bedbug (*Cimex lectularius*) has lived among humans since ancient times. These guys are small (¼ inch in length), brown, flattened, oval bugs that feed on human blood as well as animal hosts. They are sometimes mistaken for ticks. After a blood meal their bodies become swollen and more reddish in color. Bedbugs have beak-like piercing/sucking mouth parts. Females lay 1 to 12 eggs a day. The eggs are sticky and adhere to anything they touch, and in 1 to 2 weeks, they hatch and the bugs begin feeding.

Bedbugs are fast movers. Being nocturnal, they feed at night when their hosts are asleep. The person being fed on never feels the bite. It's painless. The bug injects anticoagulant-containing saliva into the host to keep the blood flowing. Adult bedbugs drink your blood for 10 to 15 minutes at a time. After feeding, they crawl away to hide in your mattress or the area surrounding your bed, until they get hungry again. Upon awakening, you will find hard, swollen, white welts on your skin, usually in rows of three or more, running along the path of blood vessels close to the surface. You may also experience severe itching that can last for several days. Scratching will only worsen the clean itching and may cause infection.

Unlike cockroaches that feed on filth, bedbugs feed on you. Therefore, even the cleanest of homes and hotels may harbor them. Usually, bedbugs hitch a ride into your house in your luggage when you return from traveling. They can also arrive via used furniture or bedding.

Bedbugs are incredibly good at hiding from you. Any sudden motion or light will send them scurrying. They like to congregate in the seams of mattresses, box springs, carpeting, and upholstery. Examine these areas thoroughly if you suspect your bedroom may be infested. You often will find black spots from their excrement where they reside. If you want to catch them in the act, take a flashlight to bed with you. Around an hour before dawn, quickly lift the covers and examine the bedding and mattress.

You may have to hire a pro to find them, and you should definitely call an exterminator to eradicate them. Sleep tight now.

What are "crabs"?

Crabs are pubic lice (*Phthirus pubis*). They are similar to the lice you find on your head, but your pubic hair is their special niche, although they can also be found on any of your body's coarse hair—armpits, eyebrows, eyelashes, beards, mustaches, and leg hair, just not the hair on top of your head. On young children, who lack pubic, leg, and facial hair, crabs go for the eyebrows and eyelashes exclusively.

How do you get them? The primary form of transmission is sexual contact. Rarely, infestation can occur through contact with another person's bedding, towel, or clothing.

How do you know if you have these little suckers (and suckers they are)? An itchy crotch is a big tip-off, as is seeing little bugs crawling around on your pubes. There are three life stages of pubic lice. The nits are lice eggs. They are about the size of this ' and hatch into nymphs, or baby lice. In a week they mature into adults that are about the size of this o, and look just like a crab that you might see on the beach. Pubic lice have six legs. Their two front legs are larger with pinchers on the end. Hence, the nickname "crabs." They must feed on human blood to survive.

Over-the-counter insecticide shampoos are available to kill crabs. After treatment, the nits can be pulled off the hair shafts with the fingernails. (Hence the term nitpicker.) Crabs in the eyebrows and eyelashes can also be removed with the fingernails or a nit comb. If the eyelashes need further treatment, a prescription ointment will be required.

Can you get maggots in your skin from a mosquito bite?

The human botfly (*Dermatobia hominis*) of South and Central America is very clever at attacking its human host. Because it would be risky to land on a person to lay its eggs directly (it might get swatted), the crafty botfly uses the mosquito as a surrogate. The female botfly grabs ahold of a female mosquito and glues her eggs onto its abdomen. The mosquito then dutifully flies to a human host and begins to feed. The heat of your body causes the botfly eggs to hatch and the larvae quickly crawl into the fresh bite wound opened by the mosquito. The yellow-brown larvae lodge themselves mouth first into your subcutaneous tissue with two tusk-like hooks. Their tail end has a tube used for breathing that they stick up like a periscope above the skin at the point of entry. As the larvae mature, they wiggle about in your skin causing considerable pain. In 8 weeks, the maggots will tire of you and drop out.

How do you get one of these rascals out of your skin? It ain't easy. There are three reported methods. First, you can use the acrid white sap of the *matatorsalo* tree (bot killer), which kills the maggot but leaves its corpse in your body. Not a great thing. Some folks put a piece of raw meat over the worm's breathing hole, in hopes it will crawl out. This method meets with varying degrees of success. The best way to get a botfly larva out of your skin, barring surgery, is to cover the burrow with glue, nail polish, mineral oil, or wax and seal this with a piece of adhesive tape. Wait 24 hours. Remove the tape and squeeze the dead bug out, like popping a zit. Some larvae will shoot across the room if squeezed out properly. (Must be quite a sight.)

If the botfly is not removed, it will grow to maturity inside you. Gross as this sounds, it may be the safest thing to do. The remedies mentioned involve the risk of leaving the dead maggot or bits of it to rot in your flesh if not completely removed. This can cause an infection worse than the problem of a bug in your flesh, depending on where that flesh might be, of course.

What kind of maggots live in the noses of sheep and goats?

Sheep and goats get something called "nose bot." Nasal botflies (*Oestrus ovis*) lay their eggs in the animal's nostrils. When the eggs hatch, the larvae crawl up the nostrils to feed. When mature, they crawl back out and drop to the ground, where they complete their development into adult flies. Infested sheep have a heavy mucus discharge that is often streaked with blood from the incisions the maggots make feeding on their sinus passages. It is estimated that up to 90 percent of sheep have had nose bots.

Caribou also get nose bots, or throat bots (*Cepehenemyia trompe*). Their little friends are deposited as maggots by the female fly on the nose of the caribou in the fall. They crawl into the animal's mouth and head for the back of the throat and sinuses. Here they spend the whole winter. In the spring they crawl out of the nose and drop to the ground. Up to 50 of these bots can overwinter in a caribou, causing the host animal to sneeze and impairing its breathing.

Another kind of botfly attacks horses. Horse bots are hairy and bee-like in appearance and are about the size of a honeybee. They lay their eggs on the legs, belly, and mane of horses. When the horse licks these eggs in the process of grooming, the eggs are ingested. The eggs then hatch inside the horse and live in its stomach. Low-level infestations will have little effect on the horse, but more severe infestations can cause problems ranging from stomach disturbances to blockage of the stomach resulting in stomach rupture. Medicines and insecticides are available from a veterinarian.

What protozoan can swim up your nose and into your brain?

This sounds like something out of a sci-fi or horror movie, but it actually happens. There's an amoeba, a unicellular blob called *Naegleria fowleri,* that attacks humans. It is commonly found in warm bodies of fresh water. Rare cases are reported each year of this amoeba entering the nose of a swimmer and traveling into the brain and spinal cord. *Naegleria* is most prone to be a problem during the hot summer months when the water is very warm and stagnant in ponds, lakes, and streams. Most people affected had been swimming underwater or diving.

You don't hear much about *Naegleria* because it rarely attacks humans; but when it does, it kills very quickly. Once in the brain, the amoeba causes brain inflammation and tissue destruction. Initial symptoms include headache, fever, nausea, vomiting, and stiff neck, followed by confusion, loss of balance, seizures, hallucinations, and death in 3 to 7 days. Although some drugs have looked promising in the laboratory, infections are almost always fatal. About 200 cases have been reported in the United States in the last 40 years, and only two people survived.

Are you worried about the remote possibility of getting this amoeba? Then avoid warm bodies of fresh water (chlorinated swimming pools are OK), don't swim underwater or dive in. If you must do so, hold your nose shut or wear one of those dorky nose clips. Good luck.

What is "delusory parasitosis"?

Some people are so paranoid about bugs on their bodies that they become psychotic. In an obsessive-compulsive disorder gone haywire, these people imagine that they are constantly under attack from invisible bugs (they happen to be right, of course). In their panic, they can scrub themselves raw and scratch themselves bloody. (I hope none of them are reading this book!) In extreme cases, sufferers have toxified their homes with pesticides, bathed themselves in gasoline, and even committed suicide.

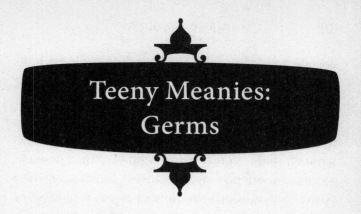

Teeny Meanies: Germs

Microbes are everywhere. Every square inch of your body surface is home to millions of these uninvited guests. While many microorganisms are very beneficial—for example, yeasts that ferment, bacteria that produce antibiotics—this chapter deals with the countless throngs of the unseen enemy that are lying in wait to sicken or kill you at any time. Germs are present all around us, on practically everything we come into contact with in our daily lives. Most of us barely give them a thought. That may prove to be a little harder for you to do after reading this chapter. *Warning:* You may not want to read on if you're germophobic!

How much bacteria is on your money?

Microbial analyses of $1 bills in western Ohio found pathogenic or potentially pathogenic microorganisms on

94 percent of them. The American Society for Microbiology studied singles collected at a high school sporting event food stand and a local supermarket in the Dayton area.[1] Of these, 59 bills carried *Staphylococcus, Streptococcus, Enterobacter, Pseudomonas,* and other pathogens that pose a risk to people with weakened immune systems. Another 5 bills bore *Staphylococcus aureus* and *Klebsiella pneumoniae,* microbes that can readily infect healthy people. *S. aureus* is found in the noses of about 25 percent of the population (so you know where their fingers have been). Only 4 bills tested clean. Talk about dirty money.

Are coins any cleaner than bills?

Coins are somewhat cleaner than paper money. Their hard, dry surfaces aren't very hospitable to bacteria. But a study that looked at quarters detected *Escherichia coli.*[2] That's the bacterium found in human waste, indicating that many of us don't practice basic bathroom hygiene. (Can you say "fecal fingers"?) Pennies seem to be the cleanest coins, their copper content having some antibacterial properties.

So should you be worried about contracting some horrible disease from your money? Not really. Most of the pathogens are present in only very low numbers, but you never know. It couldn't hurt to wash your hands after handling cash. Or you could just stick to using plastic.

In what country do they sterilize their money?

In the United States, the Federal Reserve checks cash for what they call "soil content," using machines that shine light on them to measure how much they reflect. Clean bills are shinier. About one-third of the bills tested are pulled from circulation and shredded. The Fed does a pretty good job of keeping clean-looking bills in our hands, which is good enough for most Americans.

The Japanese, however, are a little more obsessed with cleanliness, especially when it comes to their money. They don't like the thought of touching cash that has been handled by countless others with God only knows what kind of hygiene. To solve this problem, the Hitachi Company has come to the rescue with "clean" ATMs. These machines press the yens they are dispensing between rollers that are heated to 392°F for 0.1 second to sterilize them. Talk about money laundering!

Is there cocaine on your money?

Chances are good that you have cocaine-tainted money in your wallet right now. Four out of five bills in circulation at this very moment are contaminated with detectable amounts of cocaine. Lest any of you conclude that all these notes were used to snort coke or have passed through the hands of drug dealers or users, this is not the case.

Cocaine, in its powdered form, is composed of extremely fine particles. This cocaine dust, which does get on the many bills that are rolled into a tube to snort coke, is easily transferred to clean bills by money sorting and counting machines found in every bank and post office as well as ATMs. The counting machines use rollers that exert enough force on the currency to remove paper fibers from its surface, thus exposing and picking up the cocaine trapped below.

The reason American money holds on to coke is because the linen fibers it is made up of have lots of nooks and crannies in which the fine powder can lodge. The actual surface of the bills is cocaine free. Other currencies, like British paper notes, have more rounded fibers and smaller holes, which are not large enough for coke crystals to enter. Thus you will not get any detectable levels of cocaine particles on your skin from handling contaminated notes. Good to know if you are ever arrested.

A study by the Argonne National Laboratory found that the average contamination amount was 16 micrograms.[3] Not much, but enough for drug-sniffing dogs to detect. This fact has made drug prosecutions tough in court. Prosecutors used to use the presence of cocaine on bills as an excuse to confiscate the money and obtain search warrants. In view of the quantity of coke-tainted bills floating around out there, federal judges have lately ruled that the possession of tainted bills does not constitute probable cause to seize cash and launch searches. Today, judges question the admissibility of tainted cash in drug cases and must now consider the quantity of coke detected.

What's the dirtiest thing in your house?

The dirtiest room (germ-wise) is the kitchen. The dirtiest place in the kitchen is the sink. And the dirtiest thing in the whole house is the kitchen sponge. The thing that you use to clean your dishes, countertops, and table can easily harbor up to 50 million bacteria! Seeing as how food-borne bacteria are responsible for 80 million illnesses and 9,000 deaths each year in the United States, it might be a good idea to keep your sponge clean.

This isn't as simple as it sounds. Washing it out does nothing. Putting it in the dishwasher isn't much better because dishwasher water doesn't necessarily reach the 155°F needed to kill all the nasty microbes that would love to breed in your body. Some people microwave damp sponges. This may or may not be effective because microwaves have dead spots and nuking times are different for each oven. The best bet is to boil your sponge for 3 minutes or soak it in a solution of bleach and water (about a 10 percent solution will do) for 5 minutes after each use.

When wiping up countertops that may have bacteria on them, use an antibacterial spray and paper towels. Throw the towels away. You should also throw your sponges away at regular intervals, especially when they start to smell.

Does a bacterial mist shoot out of your toilet when you flush?

Dr. Charles P. Gerba, aka "Dr. Germ" (yes, he's really called that), a microbiologist at the University of Arizona, published the results of his study on toilet flushing in 1975.[4] He placed pieces of gauze in different locations around the bathroom and flushed away. He then analyzed the bacteria and viruses that landed on the gauze from the aerosol mist that emanates from johns when flushed.

Gerba found that water droplets were "going all over the place—it's like the Fourth of July."[5] An invisible cloud of microbes traveled out of the bowl for a distance of up to 8 feet. Standing near the toilet (where else are you going to stand?) while flushing can cause you to inhale this stuff. Worse yet, if your toothbrush is within 8 feet of the can, the microbial mist can land on it! The bacterial mist can hang around in the bathroom air for 2 hours after a flush.

What can you do? Put the lid down whenever you flush to reduce the aerosol plume. This, however, is impossible in public restrooms (in which case you may want to push the handle down and run like hell). Keep your toothbrush in a cover or in a drawer, or more than 8 feet from the potty. Also, don't blow you nose with the toilet paper hanging next to the bowl. It's rife with bacteria.

Gerba insists this isn't all just a ploy to get men to put

the seat down. It may be a little bit of fear-mongering though.

In case you were wondering, Gerba also has looked to see whether men's rooms or ladies' rooms were germier. Can you guess what he found? Ladies' rooms were—by far—germier than men's rooms. The places most contaminated with bacteria were, in order, the area around the sanitary napkin dispensers, the floor, and the sinks.

What are the germiest jobs?

Most of you white-collar workers out there may feel perfectly safe and secure at your desk. Truth be told, your health could be at greater risk than you may be aware. In the fall of 2005, Gerba did a study of the bacteria present on the personal office surfaces of various professions. His findings may surprise and disgust you.

Gerba's research, which was funded by the Clorox Company, examined the workspaces of nine professions for bacterial content in private offices and cubicles in Washington, DC, and Tucson, Arizona.[6] The dirtiest desktops belonged to accountants. They also had the germiest pens. It is not surprising that teachers had the germiest keyboards, mouses, and telephones. Just imagine all the grimy little fingers that touch those computers each day. The cleanest office spaces belonged to lawyers (maybe it's not such a dirty profession after all).

Surfaces regularly used by teachers, accountants, and bankers harbored from 2 to 20 times more bacteria per square inch when compared to other professions.

So, what are the germiest parts of a typical office? The telephone is totally germ-laden, followed by the desktop, water fountain handle, microwave door handle, and keyboard.[7] The area of your desk where you rest your hands has 10,000,000 bacteria! The average desktop is home to more than 400 times more bacteria than the average toilet seat! The light switch had the least amount of germs.

Why are desktops so dirty? While toilet seats get washed and disinfected regularly, desktops seldom if ever do. One reason desks are so dirty is that they are used as snack bars and lunch tables. About 57 percent of workers eat at their desks once a day. Unlike your kitchen table at home, which you probably wipe clean after each use, 75 percent of office workers say they only occasionally clean their desktops; 20 percent say they never do.

Another study compared male and female workspaces.[8] It found that the typical female workstation has 2.5 times more bacteria, mold, and yeast than a comparable male workspace. Women's desk drawers contained more food residue and thus more mold. The germiest thing in the female office was her makeup case. The germiest in the male office was his wallet.

What are the germiest public places?

The microbiologists at the University of Arizona have also studied public places to determine the germiest.[9] They found (brace yourself) frequently touched surfaces in high-traffic areas are often contaminated with bodily fluids such as blood, saliva, mucus, and sweat—all of which can carry disease-causing germs. Not to mention that they are just plain gross. After you touch these surfaces, your hands are contaminated, so you bring these nasty microbes home with you and spread them all around your house, starting with the knob on the front door and moving right on to your family.

The most germ-ridden public places are (big surprise) playgrounds and daycare centers, followed closely by buses, shopping carts (discussed in a bit), chair armrests, vending machine knobs, escalator handrails, and public phones—all the things you germophobes are terrified of.

It is interesting that some things you would think of as very germy are not. Portable public toilets were the cleanest thing on the list, probably because they are disinfected frequently. The biggest surprise, though, is the fact that an ATM machine has more germs than a public restroom door handle! This may be because people (most, one would hope) wash their hands before touching a restroom door handle, whereas no one does before using an ATM. Sounds like you should wash up after getting your cash.

The researchers used fluorescent dyes to track the germs volunteers touched in their daily routines and how they spread them throughout their homes. When those household surfaces were exposed to black lights, they "lit up like Christmas trees," according to lead researcher Kelly Reynolds.[10]

The upshot is that germophobes have a convincing case. Washing your hands several times a day makes good sense, as does disinfecting things like your telephone, doorknobs, and remote controls.

What states have enacted legislation to cut down on germy shopping carts?

One place you definitely want to be clean, but really isn't, is your supermarket. Shopping carts are veritable germ wagons. The handles are held for an average of a half hour each by a constant stream of people whose hands are covered with, for example, the blood and juices from raw meat and poultry that they have handled.[11] Add to this stew of bacteria the leaky-diapered baby bottoms that adorn the fold-down kid seats, and you've got a quite disgusting place to put your hands, not to mention your groceries.

Supermarkets are slowly beginning to realize that the bacterial zoos inhabiting their carts are a matter of public concern. Two states are enacting legislation aimed at reducing shopping-cart bacteria.

The New Jersey state legislature approved a bill in March 2007 to encourage supermarkets to provide sanitary wipes for their customers to clean the cart handle and baby seat. Arkansas, likewise, passed the Health-Conscious Shoppers Act, calling for markets to voluntarily provide sanitary wipes.[12] Perhaps in response to these laws, many supermarkets in other states are beginning to get the idea and are making sanitary wipes available to shoppers.

How germy are women's purses?

Women's purses are also collectors of bacteria. In a recent television report, a sample of 50 purses were sent to a laboratory and tested for microorganisms.[13] Almost all had bacteria. About 25 percent of the pocketbooks had *E. coli*. The report indicated that purses are set down on some very unsanitary surfaces, the worst being on the restroom floor. Other nasty resting places for pocketbooks are bus and subway floors and the aforementioned shopping carts. These bacteria are carried home on the bottom of the bags, which find themselves on countertops and tables. The report recommends wiping down purses with sanitary wipes once a day and/or just being more careful where you plop your bag.

How many people wash their hands after using a public restroom?

Infectious diseases are the number one cause of death in the world and number three in the United States. According to the Centers for Disease Control and Prevention (CDC), hand washing is the single most effective way of reducing the spread of infectious diseases.[14]

So, how many of us wash our hands after engaging in potentially dangerous activities, such as using a public restroom? Yes, research scientists have looked into this, too. In a study, conducted for the American Society for Microbiology and the Soap Detergent Manufacturers, by Harris Interactive, 6,336 individuals in four major U.S. cities were discreetly observed in public restrooms to determine their hand washing habits.[15] The study found that 91 percent of adults *claim* to wash their hands after relieving themselves in a public bathroom. If this sounds kind of high based on your own personal observations, you're right. Only 81 percent of people in the study were actually *observed* washing up. Even these numbers are believed to be high because some people may have washed their hands only because there was an observer present. We don't know what they do when they are alone. (What would you do?)

Women were found to wash their hands more often than men after using public restrooms: 90 percent versus 75 percent. (An unscientific study conducted by me found that much fewer than 75 percent of men washed their hands after urinating in a public restroom.)

The research study also found that Americans *say* that they wash their hands after using their own bathroom (83 percent of the time), before eating or handling food (77 percent), after changing a diaper (73 percent), after petting a dog or cat (42 percent), after coughing or sneezing (32 percent), and after handling money (21 percent). What do you think the *real* numbers are?

Are automatic air hand dryers more sanitary than paper towels?

Using automatic air hand dryers can actually make your hands germier than if you didn't wash them at all! Some dryers and their filters are loaded with bacteria. Rubbing your wet hands under these spreads the bacteria onto your hands. A disposable paper towel is best for drying your hands in a public restroom. It can also be used to turn off the water and open the door.

Can you get crabs from a toilet seat?

A lot of public restrooms you go into have those nice sanitary toilet seat covers. Do they do any good? If your mom was like many, she warned you of the various dangers of the public toilet seat. One was crabs—whatever they were.

Well, rest easy (or relieve yourself easy, as the case may be): Toilet seats are more innocuous than you may have thought. There are very few examples of anyone getting a disease from a toilet seat and rare instances of picking up parasites while sitting on the throne.

Most infectious sexually transmitted diseases (STDs) can't survive long on a toilet seat. About the only way you will pick up an STD on a toilet seat, is if you have unprotected sex on one. Likewise, parasites, such as crabs, don't live long away from a warm human body, and their tiny feet can't hold on to a smooth toilet seat.

So what are the toilet seat protectors for? Well, some seats, as if you needed to be told this, are quite repulsive. Instead of protecting your delicate bottom from bugs and bacteria, the covers are there to give you peace of mind and a cleaner rump. You should be much more concerned about bathroom door and faucet handles. These are crawling with germs. And if the restroom has only air hand dryers (no paper towels), you almost have to touch the doorknob unless you get rather creative in making your exit (like using your foot, shirttail, or sleeve cuffs or waiting for someone else to come in or leave).

What disease makes you bleed from *all* of your body orifices?

Maybe the most disgusting disease is Ebola—you be the judge. Ebola is a viral disease that causes a hemorrhagic fever. The Ebola virus is named for the Ebola River Valley in the Democratic Republic of the Congo, the former Zaire, in Africa. It is extremely deadly, causing pain, diarrhea, fever, vomiting, and fatigue. As the infection worsens, the sufferer experiences rashes, red eyes from bleeding arterioles, and internal and external bleeding from every imaginable hole in the body—eyes, ears, mouth, nose, anus, and penis or vagina. This is because the virus has the ability to stop the platelets from aggregating, or clotting, and to make the cell membranes permeable. Death usually occurs in 1 to 2 weeks.

The virus is thought to come from dogs or fruit bats, but no one is sure. It is spread from person to person through direct contact with infected bodily fluids. Thankfully, for the rest of the world, Ebola is limited, for the time being, to Africa because it is not readily spread through airborne transmission.

Whose peaches and ice cream dessert had a "special" surprise that infected scores of people with *Salmonella*?

If your guess is Typhoid Mary, you are definitely *Jeopardy* material! Typhoid fever is a bacterial disease caused by *Salmonella typhi*, which is spread by ingestion of food or water contaminated with human feces. It is characterized by a sustained high fever, headache, gastroenteritis, diarrhea, loss of appetite, and rose-colored rash spots. Death may follow.

The most infamous carrier of any disease is Typhoid Mary (1869–1938). Her real name was Mary Mallon and she worked as a cook in the New York City area from 1900 to 1907. Mary was a carrier of typhoid fever, showing no symptoms of the disease. She also had less-than-ideal potty habits.

In the early stages of her being a carrier, Mary was blissfully unaware of how dangerous she was. She worked as a cook for several different families. Many members of each household came down with typhoid fever. Mary was involved in trying to nurse them back to health, which only made things worse. In a span of 7 years, she infected at least seven households, sickening 22 people, one of whom died. Apparently, the dish that did people in was Mary's signature dessert—peaches and ice cream . . . with a little added surprise.

The landlord of one of the houses with sick people called in an investigator, who suspected Mary was responsible. When he approached her, Mary refused to give the investigator a sample of her stool and urine. She vehemently sent him packing. Mary did not believe she could have a disease if she showed no symptoms. Finally, the New York City Department of Health detained Mary and found her to be a carrier. She was subsequently quarantined for 3 years, after which time they agreed to free Mary if she promised not to work with food anymore. Bad plan! Instead, they should have taught her to wash her hands after taking a dump.

In 1925, pigheaded Mary changed her name to Mary

Brown (how apropos) and went right back to serving up her special "fecal-surprise" dishes. This time, Mary chose to cook for New York's Sloan Hospital. She proceeded to infect 25 more people, 2 of whom died. Finally, Mary was detained and isolated for the rest of her life. She died of pneumonia at the age of 69. Upon autopsy, it was discovered that her gallbladder was loaded with S. typhi!

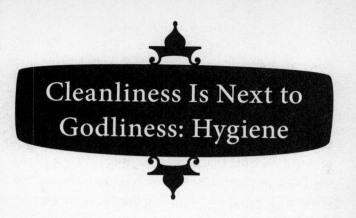

Cleanliness Is Next to Godliness: Hygiene

For the vast majority of human history, personal hygiene was almost nonexistent. It is only within about the last century or so that people had any idea that filth and human waste lead to sickness and death. The germ theory was unknown, and our ancestors lived in ignorance of the deadly consequences of their lack of hygiene. After a brief period of relative cleanliness in ancient Greece and Rome, the world fell into the Dark Ages (or what I like to call the "Dirty Stinky Ages"). People wore dirt with pride and most never had a bath in their lives!

Has it ever been illegal to take a bath?

The Romans' obsession with baths and bathing is well documented. After the fall of the Roman Empire, however, the world entered the Dark Ages. During this period, hygiene was basically unknown in the Western world. In a radically foul move away from the excesses of the Roman baths, early Christian leaders decided that cleanliness was not next to godliness. St. Francis of Assisi declared that an unwashed body was a stinking badge of piety.[1] Monks, however, were allowed the occasional cold bath when impure thoughts entered their heads.

Even royalty eschewed bathing. Queen Isabella of Castile once bragged that she only had two baths in her life: one when she was born and one before her wedding. The Puritans in Colonial America saw bathing as immoral because it involved nudity and, therefore, would lead to hanky-panky. Pennsylvania and Virginia both had laws on the books prohibiting or severely limiting bathing. In early Philadelphia, one could be jailed for such an outrageous activity.

In Europe, no such laws were needed. Bathing really wasn't an option for most folks. Clean water was not to be found. There was no public water supply, and most lakes and rivers were polluted and cold. In England, soap was considered a luxury and was taxed at a rate of 100 percent, making it available only to the affluent. By the nineteenth century, both Europeans and urban Americans were living in a world of filth. People actually believed that a nice thick layer of dirt protected them from disease.

When did entire families have to share the same bathwater?

In the days of our great unwashed past, only the rich could afford an occasional hot bath. There was one catch, however: Everyone in the house had to use the same water. The male head of household had dibs on being first. His tub was full of nice, clean hot water. When he was done, the other males of the house took their turns, followed by the females and finally by the young. As you may well imagine, the water got colder and filthier with each subsequent bath. By the time the youngest members of the home got in, the water was so dirty as to be a joke. When everyone was finished bathing, it was time to empty the tub. People quipped that the water was so dirty that it should first be checked to see if anyone had been forgotten in there, giving rise to the expression "Don't throw the baby out with the bathwater."

Why did some people in France protest when defecating in the streets was outlawed?

In 1831, England experienced its first cholera outbreak. The disease traveled to America with immigrants who had been packed into the hold of a ship, where they were forced to share slop buckets and dirty water; sanitation practices in early American cities weren't much better.

People had no idea about what diseases were or how they spread. Thus encouraging more hygienic practices was difficult. For instance, when Milwaukee tried to clean up the garbage that clogged the city, the "rag pickers" and "swill children," who eked out a living removing vile matter from the streets, revolted. In France, people used to defecating in the streets protested its banning, claiming that their ancestors had defecated there, so it was their God-given right.

In the United States, the first city to introduce piped water was Philadelphia, in 1802. By 1860, 136 cities had piped water systems. With piped water available, per capita water use skyrocketed from 3 gallons per person per day to 30 to 50 gallons per person per day. Levels of personal hygiene also soared, and the incidence of water-borne diseases, such as cholera, fell. However, cities that drew their water supply from rivers downstream from sewer discharges began suffering from typhoid outbreaks.

Does taking a bath leave you with a film of slime?

What do you think gets you cleaner, a bath or a shower? This is a tricky question. Baths are more deep cleaning, but you end up in a pool of your own dirt. Showers rinse the dirt down the drain but get you less clean. To get really clean, you need to remove oil, dirt, and flakes of old skin. You can scrub with a loofah all you want in the shower; but to properly exfoliate dead skin cells, you need to first hydrate the skin. This takes soaking. Soapy water acts as a surfactant, reducing the surface tension of the water, allowing it to penetrate deeper into the skin. The skin flakes will then float away.

The gross problem with bathing is that you are left in a pool of dead skin, oil, dirt, and grime that's bound to the soap floating on top of the water. When you stand up, you are coated with a film of this slime. The solution to getting really clean is taking a quick shower before getting out of the tub.

By the by, the average American spends 11 minutes in the shower and about 20 minutes in the tub and claims to bathe or shower at least seven times a week.

What company has collected 18,000 samples of sweat?

Human sweat is, in and of itself, odorless. Bacteria use the warmth and moisture found in the underarms to ferment sweat into stinky compounds. Underarm hair adds to the smell because it increases the surface area available for the bacteria to grow on. There are three ways to reduce body odor (BO)—reduce moisture, kill bacteria, or use perfumes to mask the smell.

Deodorants are usually alcohol based, which helps them kill bacteria. Many contain antimicrobials. They often are combined with an antiperspirant, such as aluminum chlorohydrate, aluminum chloride, or aluminum zirconium, to reduce the moisture available for bacterial growth. Aluminum compounds react with the electrolytes in sweat to form a gel that plugs the ducts of the sweat glands, thus preventing sweating. The best antiperspirants block only about 60 percent of sweat. They are really designed to reduce just underarm sweat. They should never be applied all over your body because this will cause you to overheat. Over time, the plugs are removed by the natural sloughing off of skin.

The first commercially available deodorant was Mum, introduced in 1888, by a long-forgotten Philadelphia inventor. The first roll-on deodorant was Ban Roll-On, which debuted in 1952. It was inspired by the invention of the ballpoint pen.

The Unilever Company keeps a database of 18,000 samples of sweat from consumers who are tested for antiperspirant effectiveness. The volunteers are put in a room that is heated to 100°F with a relative humidity of 35 percent. Once good and sweaty, their perspiration is collected. (There's great job for you.)

What did people use before toilet paper?

Whatever was on hand. (Sorry.) What would *you* use if there were no paper? That's what they used: leaves, grass, corncobs, shells, rocks. Well, you get the idea. There weren't a lot of good options.

Ancient Romans used a sponge on the end of a stick that was kept in a jar of salty water. (This is the origin of the expression "Getting the wrong end of the stick.") The Roman method was better than that of the ancient Greeks, who used stones and pieces of clay. Arabs just used their left hand and water (Eew!), which is why the left hand is still considered unclean in many Arab cultures. This practice may also explain why we greet people by shaking the right hand. Eskimos used snow and moss. (Brrr!) Hawaiians used coconut shells. Vikings used old bits of wool. Spanish and Portuguese sailors used the frayed ends of anchor rope. French royalty used lace. Happily, for most of us today, our only decision is one ply or two.

Did early mass-produced toilet paper give you splinters?

Paper that was specifically made for wiping one's bottom appeared in China in the late 1300s. The emperor ordered some up in 2-foot by 3-foot squares. No chintzy little one-ply squares for him. The idea doesn't seem to have spread to the outside world for centuries.

It wasn't until 1857, for example, that toilet paper appeared in America. Before that (and for some time thereafter), corncobs, the Sears & Roebuck Catalog, and the *Old Farmer's Almanac* served the purpose. (The almanac even had a hole in the upper corner for hanging it in the outhouse.) It was in that fateful year that Joseph C. Gayetty introduced Gayetty's Medicated Paper, the first packaged toilet paper. The paper was premoistened and medicated with aloe and had his name emblazoned on every sheet. It was sold in pharmacies.

The first perforated toilet paper was sold by the Albany Perforated Wrapping Paper Company in 1877. Scott Paper put perforated paper on a roll in 1879. They were too embarrassed, however, to put their name on it. Toilet paper was a taboo subject back then, so they put the names of industrial customers on instead, one being the Waldorf Hotel, which led to the popular Waldorf brand.

In 1935, Northern Tissue advertised their paper as "splinter free." That's right, *splinter free*. You see, early paper production sometimes left splinters embedded in the paper. Talk about a pain in the butt!

Two-ply paper from St. Andrew's Paper Mill in England debuted in 1942. Around that time softer, more pliable toilet paper became available. For most of the twentieth century, one could buy hard or soft toilet paper. The hard paper was shiny on one side and much cheaper. The price of soft paper has come way down; and today, soft paper is ubiquitous. Much to the delight of derrieres everywhere!

Would you like to know the results of the great toilet paper survey?

Bet you didn't know there was such a thing. Actually, a compilation of several surveys indicates the following about our toilet paper usage:

- 49 percent of people say that, after food, they would pick TP as the next most important thing to have on a desert island.

- 40 percent of wipers like to wad up the paper; 40 percent are folders; and 20 percent wrap it around their hand. Men are more likely to be folders, women crumplers.

- The average wiper uses 8.6 sheets per visit and around 56 per day. Annually, that adds up to 20,805 sheets. That's a lot of sheet.

- Johnny Carson created a toilet paper shortage in 1973, when on *The Tonight Show* he cracked that the United States was facing a toilet paper shortage. The next day, millions of people ran out and bought up all the TP they could get their hands on.

Why do we call the toilet a "john"?

Perhaps the one modern convenience we most take for granted is the toilet. It wasn't until very recently that the flush toilet entered our homes. The ancient Romans created the first sophisticated water supply and sewer systems. The Roman toilet, like those in many countries of the Far East today, consisted of an oblong hole in the floor, without a seat, over a sewer. The toilet never really caught on though. While the rich in some cultures enjoyed its benefits, the vast majority of the world's population did not. In the absence of toilets and indoor plumbing, people urinated and defecated wherever they could—on the side of the road, in a river, behind a bush.

The first water closet resembling today's toilet was created for Queen Elizabeth I by her godson, Sir John Harington, in 1596. Too far ahead of its time, the invention was ridiculed by society, and Harington made no more, although the queen was said to have loved hers. We still honor Harington for his invention whenever we say we have to go to the john. It was 200 years before another inventor would reinvent the water closet (toilet), but it was not until 1775 that a patent for a flushing toilet was issued to Alexander Cummings. Countless other inventors and innovations would occur before the toilet we know today would come into wide use.

Didn't Thomas Crapper invent the toilet?

As any trivia buff worth his salt knows, this is not the case. However, Thomas Crapper (1836–1910) was in fact a real person. He was an English plumber and even held patents for improvements to water closets, drain systems, manhole covers, and pipe joints. The toilet had been around for some time before Crapper got into the plumbing game. He even served as the royal sanitary engineer; but alas, he did not invent the toilet.

We call toilets crappers because during World War I, the American doughboys in England saw the words "T. Crapper—Chelsea" printed on toilet tanks and took to calling them "crappers."

So where does the word *crap* come from? This one has nothing to do with Thomas Crapper. No one is sure, but the word *crap* probably comes from the Dutch *krappe* and the German *krape,* meaning "a vile and inedible fish."

When were city streets covered in excrement?

Up until the end of the nineteenth century, only the well-to-do in Europe had toilets or any kind of indoor plumbing. Since time immemorial, folks kept chamber pots by their beds, which they simply dumped out the window. During the period of the Industrial Revolution, there was a tremendous growth of tenements and slums. Chamber pot droppings fouled every square inch of city sidewalks and streets. There were also vast quantities of horse manure clogging the byways. Community pits, called cesspools, were introduced as common depositories for human waste. Night men had the odious job of climbing into these slop pits and shoveling out their contents into barrels. Those with greater resources may have had an outhouse or latrine. Dry latrines were emptied by menial laborers using buckets. They became known as the "bucket brigade."

Castles of old had their version of the cesspool. They called it a moat. That's right. The actual presence of pools of water that surrounded fortified structures did little to slow a determined enemy down, but their contents may have.

What cultures wash their bottoms with a pot of water after relieving themselves?

Unless you are Muslim, Middle Eastern, or South Asian, you probably don't know. *Lota* is a Hindi or Urdu word for "pot." It generally refers to a pot with a handle and a spout that is used to pour water on one's anus for the purpose of cleaning up after defecation. Cleaning is facilitated by holding the lota in the right hand, pouring water on the nether regions, and cleaning down there with the left hand. Bidets have begun to replace the lota in more affluent homes.

So, what *is* a bidet?

Many North Americans seem somewhat confused by the bidet and aren't sure what to do on one. Is it a urinal? Is it just for women?

In European countries like Greece, Italy, Portugal, and Spain; South American countries like Argentina and Uruguay; parts of Asia and especially India; and many Middle Eastern countries, bidets are a common bathroom fixture that people cannot live without. In fact, residents of these countries think that just wiping yourself with dry toilet paper after going is quite disgusting. They are at odds as to what to do when traveling to "backward" nations like the United States, where the hotels don't have bidets. Many foreign visitors are reduced to using the showerhead or bathtub. The idea of having intercourse with someone who hasn't used a bidet disgusts them.

Thought to have originated in France around 1710, the word *bidet* is French for "pony." This makes sense, for one mounts and "rides" a bidet much like a pony.

Bidets are used to wash the anus and genitals after going to the bathroom. They can also be used for cleaning the feet, or for a baby bath, although this is not recommended. You do not urinate or defecate in a bidet; this is done in the toilet. The bidet is used to wash up afterward.

One sits facing the tap end to clean the genitals and facing backward to wash the anus. Some bidets shoot an arc of water into the air and some have a warm water tap that can be used to fill the basin for washing. Bidet users generally use toilet paper first, as Americans do, then head to the bidet. After washing, the bottom is dried with toilet paper or a special towel that is changed daily.

What are "paperless toilets"?

Toilets can also be outfitted with bidet nozzles. These are popular in Japan and are called "paperless toilets," "bidet toilets," or "Washlets." Introduced in 1980, Washlets are now found in about 60 percent of Japanese households. They are the state of the art in bathroom hygiene. When a user approaches, the Washlet automatically opens the lid. Through a number of pulsating and massaging functions, the water jets wash the anus and vulva, dry them afterward with warm air, flush, and close the lid, all automatically. (This all sounds a bit like something from *The Jetsons,* but it allows the user more time to do the crossword and also provides a cleaner tuchus than the average barbaric American's.)

Can you handle some more toilet trivia?

The first stall in a restroom is said to be the cleanest. Apparently many people skip it, erroneously thinking that it is the most used and, therefore, the dirtiest.

Astronauts strap themselves onto a toilet seat that forms an airtight seal on their bottom. A vacuum sucks up their poop so it doesn't go floating about the cabin. Urine is recycled into drinking water on long space trips.

What did women use before sanitary napkins?

Well, just as with toilet paper, use your imagination. Anything that was available was put to use. Folded old rags were a particular favorite for ages. Hence the euphemism "on the rag." Before disposable napkins, women of means would reuse cotton pads after washing.

The first disposable sanitary napkins appeared in

Germany in the 1880s, but were not available in America till later. Tampons first became available in the 1920s, but didn't gain wide acceptance until the 1940s.

When did people start wearing underwear?

Underwear—we all take it for granted. However, it is a rather recent article of clothing. In the days of yore, people didn't wear any. Even noblewomen, who wore corsets and petticoats, didn't wear anything between their legs.

Yes, our ancestors were an unsanitary lot. Because few had access to clean water, the laundering of clothing was almost nonexistent. The vast majority of the filthy masses wore the same clothes for up to a year, unwashed. Imagine what a stinking mess underpants would have quickly become! One's privates would have been a breeding ground for all sorts of nasty infections. A vagina or penis exposed to the air, however, might not have been fresh as a daisy but would stay drier, cooler, and less hospitable to germ growth.

There was another advantage to women going *au naturel*. It simplified the act of relieving oneself. All a lady had to do was find a convenient spot and squat. Panties would have complicated things somewhat.

In colder climates, undergarments may have been worn to provide warmth. They usually were in the form of tights, stockings, or tunics.

Why did Tudor women blacken their teeth?

During the reign of Henry VIII, sugar was the newest food craze in Europe. It was considered exotic, and it was very expensive. Only the wealthy could afford it. Affluent Tudor people soon came to realize that there was a bigger price to pay for their love of sugar than just money. Sugar made their teeth rot and turn black. Even Queen Elizabeth had black teeth. Because she was the fashion trendsetter of her age, other women followed her royal example. Many women, especially those too poor to buy lots of sugar, actually blackened their teeth to appear wealthy and more like the queen.

What animal's penis bone was once used as a toothpick?

Before the toothbrush was invented, ancients used "chewing sticks." As early as the Babylonians in 3500 BCE, people chewed on pieces of wood about the size of a pencil. Sticks were selected from aromatic trees that would freshen the breath. One end was chewed until it became softened and brush-like, while the other was shaped into a point and used for picking crud out from between the teeth. People have most likely been picking their teeth with toothpicks since time immemorial. Among the items commonly used were bird feathers, animal bones, twigs, porcupine quills, and somewhat repulsively, a raccoon baculum, or the little bone from the raccoon penis. (*Note:* More Americans choke to death each year on toothpicks than any other object.)

The actual bristle toothbrush first appeared in seventeenth-century China. Englishman William Addis is credited with creating the first mass-produced toothbrush. Its handle was carved from cattle bone, with bristles plucked from the shoulder and neck of swine. Before Addis, Europeans had been cleaning their teeth by rubbing a rag on them. Nylon bristles first appeared in 1938.

Most Americans didn't start brushing their teeth until after World War II. This is one case of a terrible war having some positive repercussions. The U.S. Army forced its soldiers to brush their teeth daily, and the GIs brought this new habit back home with them. Others soon followed suit.

Mao Tse-tung bragged that he never brushed his teeth, citing the fact that tigers don't brush their teeth as his rationale.

Does bad breath come from the same chemical compounds found in corpses?

Halitosis is a word meaning "bad breath." The makers of the antiseptic Listerine seized on the name in their 1922 "Even Your Best Friend Won't Tell You" advertising campaign, making it a household word.

Some bad breath is caused by the food you eat—things like garlic and onions—and is temporary. Your digestive system breaks these foods down into their component molecules, some of which are quite odoriferous. These are absorbed into the bloodstream and some find their way to the lungs, where they are exhaled. In a day or so, these compounds dissipate and the odor goes away.

For the majority of the 85 to 90 percent of people who have more permanent bad breath, the cause is the bacteria that live in their mouths. Bacteria, like other living things, consume foods and excrete wastes. These wastes, in the form of sulfur compounds, usually are at the root of your breath odors. Sulfur compounds also create the stink associated with stables, rotten eggs, and the ocean. Dentists refer to these chemicals as "volatile sulfur compounds" (VSCs).

Your oral bacteria produce some other nasty waste products with wicked odors, including the following:

- *Cadaverine:* as the name implies, the smell given off by corpses
- *Isovaleric acid:* the stinky feet smell
- *Putrescine:* the chemical that gives rotten meat its stench
- *Skatole:* the smell of feces

Every one of us has a mix of these unsavory chemicals in our mouths. Is it any wonder that so many people have bad breath?

How can you tell if you have bad breath?

Unless you have kids or a spouse, who usually aren't shy about pointing out such things, you may not be sure. Friends and coworkers may be loath to bring up this delicate subject, even though they may be dying to do so. If you have a bad taste in your mouth you probably have bad breath. There are a couple of at home tests you can try.

Lick the back of your wrist with your tongue and let it dry. A quick sniff will tell you if you have any stinky bacteria on the front of your tongue. Because most of the really obnoxious smells come from the back of your tongue, another test is needed. Take an inverted tea-spoon and scrape the top of your tongue as far back as you can without gagging. You should see a thick whit-ish material on the spoon. This is plaque. Take a whiff. This is what your companions smell every time you open your mouth. You can also sample your breath by wearing a cheap dust mask for a few minutes.

It's the bacteria that live in the plaque layer on your tongue that cause most bad breath problems. This layer is a perfect home for anaerobic bacteria (bacteria that grow without oxygen). Stick out your tongue and look in the mirror. See that whitish layer on top? That's plaque. It should get thicker and whiter the farther back on your tongue you look. This is because the front of your tongue rubs up against the top of your mouth, which scrapes it away. The back of your tongue rarely touches the roof of the mouth, so the plaque there doesn't get rubbed off. It's this thick layer at the back that really reeks.

Different people have different kinds of tongue-surface textures and different kinds of plaque layers. Some folks have deeply grooved or furrowed tongues. These collect more stuff than will a smoother tongue. A dental plaque layer the thickness of a piece of paper is enough to create an oxygen-depleted environment that will promote the growth of anaerobic bacteria.

So, how can you get rid of plaque? A couple of options exist. The simplest is gently brushing your tongue when you brush your teeth. A more thorough cleaning can be achieved by using a teaspoon or a tongue scraper. This is a device with a plastic or metal loop at one end that you use to scrape plaque from the surface of your tongue. They have been around, in one form or another, since the days of ancient China.

Breath fresheners and gums won't do anything but mask your bad breath for a short time. Antiseptic mouthwashes will kill bacteria and lead to longer relief.

What professional gets paid to smell your bad breath?

OK, so you've figured out that you have bad breath. Can you seek professional help? Yes, and he or she will want to quantify just how wicked your breath is by conducting scientific tests.

The first test, which isn't so scientific, is called an

organoleptic test. Simply put, the health-care professional smells your breath. (Great job.) Dentists conduct
this test on a daily basis. It's very good, because the
human nose can detect up to 10,000 different smells.
This test, however, is not scientifically objective and
can't be quantified.

Many dentists use a device called a halimeter. These
machines were introduced in 1991 and measure the
level of VSCs in your breath. A high level of VSCs indicates stinky breath.

To determine exactly which VSCs are in your breath,
a gas chromatography test can be conducted. This test is
used infrequently because it is lengthy, expensive, and
requires specially trained technicians.

What causes "morning breath"?

Even if you are not prone to bad breath, yours will still
smell kind of funky when you wake up in the morning. Morning breath is a result of a dry mouth. When
you sleep, your salivary glands reduce their production
of saliva. Why does a dry mouth smell? One answer is
that your spit helps cleanse the mouth. It contains antibiotics and antimicrobials that kill many of the nasty,
stinky germs that live there. During the night, these
little guys can flourish. You also swallow less in your
sleep. Swallowing takes away a lot of these bacteria and
their wastes.

Some people have chronically dry mouths. This

condition is called "xerostomia." It can be a side effect of many different medications. Also, as people age, their salivary glands don't function as effectively. People who are very nervous or talk a lot are also prone to dry mouth.

When did diners wipe their greasy fingers on their hair?

When you are invited to someone's house for dinner, you expect that napkins will be supplied. This was not the case for much of human history. In the old days, before utensils appeared at the table, people ate with their fingers. In Roman times, the host supplied one napkin for his guests to tie around the neck to catch falling food, and the guests brought one of their own to wrap up any leftovers to take home. By the Middle Ages, napkins had fallen from favor. If the host did not provide them, guests wiped their hands on the tablecloth, if there was one, or on their clothes or hair!

In what country is spitting in public socially acceptable?

By the mid-1800s, chewing tobacco was a favorite pastime. The only problem was that chewers felt they had the God-given right to spit their disgusting tobacco juice wherever they wanted, be they indoors or out. Sidewalks, streets, hotel and bank lobbies, and virtually any other public surface were covered with hideous, brown spit. Happily, spittoons, also known as cuspidors, which had been used in Southeast Asia for centuries, found their way into the United States and England by 1840.

A spittoon is a flat-bottomed, weighted pot with a wide flange around the top. They are commonly made of brass, but can also be found in porcelain. Some have drain holes in the bottom to facilitate cleaning. They became ubiquitous fixtures in all public places; even railway cars and churches had them. All fine homes had one in each room. Gentlemen prided themselves on their spitting prowess. The word *pinger* was coined for the sound an accurate gob of tobacco made when it hit the side of a metal spittoon.

The public was concerned about the spread of tuberculosis (TB), a leading killer of the time. Getting the hardcore spitters to use spittoons was no easy task. The Boy Scouts had campaigns to post "Do Not Spit on the Sidewalk" signs on city streets. Spittoons were filled with the antiseptic carbolic acid to kill germs. TB sufferers were encouraged to carry mini cuspidors in their pockets that they could spit into. TB patients today do the same thing.

After the 1918 flu pandemic, there was even more pressure to eliminate spittoons and chewing tobacco. Chewing gum began to catch on with the younger crowd and cigarettes gained in popularity. At the outset of World War II, many brass cuspidors ended up recycled as scrap for the war effort.

While public spitting is now considered bad form in the United States, in places like China, men and women have no compunction about letting a loogie fly wherever they happen to be. It is common for beautiful floors in banks and stores to be littered with disgusting gobs of white mucus.

FYI: The record for tobacco spitting is 53 feet 3 inches, set in 1997.

Did anyone ever have pubic hair down to his or her knees?

For most of us, pubic hair growth is determinate. This means that it grows to a predetermined length and stops. Kind of like leg or armpit hair. Male facial hair and the hair on our heads is indeterminate, meaning it can keep on growing. For some, pubic hair is indeterminate. As reported in *The Illustrated Book of Sexual Records,* one woman had pubic hair down to her knees![2] Another woman's bush was so thick and full that it went almost up to her belly button in front and several inches up her buttocks in the back.

What are some other hair-raising records?

Voluminous ear hair also grosses out many people. We tend to think of this as an old man's condition. There's one guy in India who is cited as having the world's longest ear hair, according to the good folks at Guinness World Records.[3] His name is Radhakant Bajpai, and his ear locks can be pulled out to a length of 13.2 centimeters (5.19 inches). He smashed the record of Indian Antony Victor: 11.5 centimeters. Another Indian guy, B. D. Tyagi of Bhopal, India, has ear hair 10.2 centimeters long. (There must be something in the water in India.)

While we are on the subject of long hair, a guy in New York State has eyebrow hair 3 inches long! (Guess he never heard of tweezers.) The longest beard belonged to Hans Langseth of Norway. At his death, in 1927, it measured 17½ feet long. The longest beard on a woman belonged to Vivian Wheeler of Wood River, Illinois. It measured 11 inches! The longest head of hair is on a Chinese woman named Xie Qiuping; it measured 18 feet 5 inches in 2004.

When did people wear cones of grease on their heads?

It was the fashion around 1400 BCE for wealthy Egyptian women to wear cones of scented grease on top of their heads while attending banquets. As the party wore on, the heat from the head slowly melted the grease, which would run down the head and body, covering the skin in an oily sheen and making the clothes wonderfully cool and fragrant. Sounds divine.

When did women have vermin in their hairdos?

Before the time of Louis XV of France, there was no such thing as a beauty salon or hairdresser. Up until that time, women of means wore wigs to achieve their coiffure. Louie's mistress, Madame Pompadour, changed all that.

The French court began to throw elaborate theme parties. Noblewomen hired artists to create hairstyles for them that fit in with the theme of the party. The hair was draped over a frame and cemented with a paste that hardened it in place. The hairdo was then powdered and decorated with all manner of objects, such as live birds in cages, waterfalls, and naval battles. The word *hairdresser* comes from these artists who "dressed" the hair with ornamentation. In 1762, there were no hairdressers in Paris; 5 years later, there were more than 1,200.

One little problem with these massive hairdos was that bear grease and beef lard were often used to hold them together. Because they were somewhat expensive, women wanted to keep the hairstyles for a week or two. The grease and lard, as you can imagine, began to get putrid after a few days, which tended to attract vermin to the ladies' hair as they slept! This is how the term *rat's nest* came to mean "messy hair."

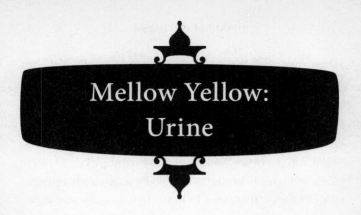

Mellow Yellow: Urine

We all urinate several times a day (or at least we should). For some reason, most people find pee to be somehow impure and repulsive. Heaven forbid you get a drop of this terrible stuff on your hands while relieving yourself! They must be quickly sanitized. You may be surprised to learn that fresh urine is completely sterile. Some people even drink pee. Over the years, urine has been used for lots of other purposes, many of which will make you cringe.

Can you drink your urine?

OK, so maybe this isn't something that you're ever going to do, but just imagine you are marooned on a desert island waiting for rescue with nothing to drink. Just so you know, yes, you can drink your urine; although, because it's saline, it won't rehydrate you much better than seawater. Some people actually enjoy drinking their own pee. We'll get to that later. For now, let's see what urine is.

Along with being salty, urine is also slightly acidic. Pee is 95 percent water and has an ammonia-like odor due to the nitrogenous wastes (and other stuff) that make up the other 5 percent. It also contains dead blood cells and other material the body wants to eliminate. The kidneys filter the blood plasma, allowing water, sugars, vitamins, amino acids, and other vital substances to remain in the bloodstream. They eliminate any excess amounts of these substances as well as urea from protein digestion, uric acid, creatinine from muscle breakdown, hormone waste, and toxins. Fresh urine is sterile when it leaves the body. This watery solution of metabolic wastes, dissolved salts, and organic materials is stored in the bladder until it is eliminated through the urethra.

The average adult urinates between 1 and 2 quarts a day. Your first morning pee will be the most concentrated. The more you drink, the more diluted it becomes, and the lighter its color.

Pee is one of the only sterile things in the body; the others are blood, the solid organs, and the cerebrospinal fluid. The only "toxic" component in urine is the urea, but there isn't enough quantity to cause you much trouble. However, drinking another person's pee may be more problematic. Theoretically, any of numerous infections (hepatitis B, chlamydia, herpes, etc.) could be transmitted to you by swallowing another's urine. (Medical science hasn't devoted much time to the matter, as yet.)

Having said this, there are plenty of people around the world who drink urine on a daily basis.

Why *do* some people drink urine?

Although many of us find this practice repellant (even on a desert island), more than 3 million Chinese drink their own urine in the belief that it is good for them. Indian holy men have been quaffing the stuff for millennia. Mahatma Gandhi is said to have started each day with a nice warm cup of his urine.

There's also something called "urine therapy." It is thought to prevent sickness, cure disease, enhance beauty, and even cleanse the bowels! To obtain its curative and preventative benefits, most practitioners of urine therapy like to drink from the midstream of their morning flow. Some enjoy it piping hot, straight from the source. Others mix it with juice or serve it over fruit.

Gargling with wee to which saffron has been added is practiced to soothe throat infections. A few drops in the eyes and ears can keep them healthy and happy. For beauty enhancement, women wash with it. Some Japanese ladies bathe in urine to improve their skin quality. And hardcore pee worshipers enjoy a good urine enema or douche.

Followers of urine therapy claim that urine contains compounds that are very specific to the individual from which it comes. It is antibacterial, antifungal, antiviral, antineoplastic (anticancer), anticonvulsive, and anti-spasmodic. Many of the so-called waste products found in urine are simply nutrients and chemicals that the body did not need at the time they passed through the kidneys. Drinking it gives the body another chance to make use of these compounds.

Still having doubts? Urine therapy devotees believe that Solomon recommends drinking your own pee in the Bible: "Drink waters from thy own cistern, flowing water from thy own well" (Proverbs 5:15). (Of course, biblical scholars will tell you this passage actually warns against the evils of adultery.)

How is urine used in religious ceremonies?

Various peoples also drink urine for religious reasons. Certain Hindus practice a tantric religious rite called *amaroli*. Because urine comes from the same orifice as semen, there seems to be some connection with pee as a sexual energizer.

Siberian tribesmen made a broth from fly agaric mushrooms that they drank to achieve spiritual enlightenment while hallucinating. Mushrooms are hard to find in Siberia during the cold months and often were in short supply. Because much of the psychedelic drug passes through the body in the urine, drinking it can produce another high. Siberians who were unfortunate enough not to have had any mushrooms of their own to trip on would collect the pee of those who did and thus could experience a pretty doggone good trip themselves.

Why did doctors used to taste a patient's urine?

There isn't enough HMO money around for a modern physician to sip your urine. Back in the days before the big bucks, however, doctors really earned their pay when treating diabetics.

One unique side effect of diabetes is that it makes your pee taste sweet. Ancient Arab, Hindu, and Chinese texts make mention of this phenomenon. The first modern physician to make this connection was an English doctor named Thomas Willis, in 1674. It's not clear what gave him the idea to taste urine, but once he tried diabetic urine he apparently enjoyed it, having stated that it was "wonderfully sweet, as if it were imbued with honey or sugar." Until more recent tests for blood and urine sugars were developed, doctors tasted pee to help diagnose diabetes. Talk about upholding the Hippocratic oath!

What can turn your urine blue?

Talk about unsettling—imagine looking down while peeing to find blue urine coming out! The normal color range of urine (as if you need to be told this) is anywhere from light yellow to dark amber. One of the things eliminated in your pee is urochrome, which is a yellow pigment that comes from the processing of dead blood cells in the liver. Urochrome gives urine its yellow color. Your pee can become deep yellow if you have been sweating a lot or have not been drinking enough liquids.

Under certain conditions, however, any number of unusual colors are possible. The following is a list of possible urine colors and what each may indicate:

- *Blue/Green:* The main culprit in cases of blue or green urine is the dye methylene blue. It is found in certain medications, such as Trac Tabs and Uroblue. These are taken to help reduce bladder inflammation or irritation. Many multivitamins can impart a bluish hue to your urine. If you are not taking medications or vitamins, your blue pee may be caused by the bacterium *Pseudomonas.*

- *Orange:* Drugs such as phenazopyridine (Pyridium), ethoxazene (Serenium), rifampin, phenacetin, and sulfasalazine can make your pee orange, as can vitamin C, riboflavin, and even carrots.

- *Brown/Black:* People with melanoma may excrete melanin and melanogen in their urine. Brown or black urine can also occur with copper or phenol poisoning. One less worrisome reason your pee may be brownish black is the consumption of large amounts of rhubarb, fava beans, or aloe.

- *White:* White or cloudy urine most commonly indicates excess phosphate crystals in your pee. Called phosphaturia, it can result after drinking copious amounts of milk. White urine may also be caused by white blood cells from a urinary tract infection.

- *Clear:* If you have been drinking lots of water or diuretics like caffeine or beer, your pee will have little or no color.

- *Red/Pink:* One common cause of red urine is beets. Their deep red coloration comes from the pigment betacyanin. Most people can metabolize this pigment and pass it normally through their bodies. The ability to metabolize it is controlled by a recessive gene. Those who have two recessive genes cannot metabolize betacyanin. The pigment leaves the body in the urine, which it colors bright red. Red or pink urine may also indicate a serious medical problem, which should prompt an immediate visit to your doctor. The reddish color may be from red blood cells (blood) and usually is a sign of some underlying medical problem.

How much urine can your bladder hold?

Urine is made in the kidneys. Every minute, a quart of blood passes through them in the renal arteries. The waste products in your blood are removed in the form of urine. It drips from the kidneys through the ureters into the bladder, a balloon-like sack. Just like a balloon, your bladder is shriveled up when it is empty. It can expand enough to hold about 2 cups of pee. When it is full, the bladder sends a message to the brain telling it so. Then the bladder loosens a ring of muscle around the hole at its base, the internal sphincter. Fortunately, there is another ring, the external sphincter, below the first, that is controlled by the brain, or else you'd need to wear diapers. Holding this second ring shut is a learned skill. This is why babies need to be potty trained. Problems with the external sphincter lead to incontinence. When all systems are go, muscles that line the bladder will contract, sending forth the golden stream. Ahhh . . .

As just noted, the bladder can hold about 2 cups of urine; however, you will start to feel the urge to pee when around ½ cup has accumulated.

What infection can be cured by peeing in the shower?

Athlete's foot (tinea pedis) is a foot infection caused by one of the following parasitic fungi—*Trichophyton rubrum, Trichophyton interdigitale,* or *Epidermophyton floccosum.* The infection loves warm, damp, dark places, like the spaces between your toes. It also persists for long periods of time in the environment, which is why it is so easy to catch in communal places like locker-room showers. Symptoms of athlete's foot are itchy, flaking, scaling skin. You may also experience blistered and cracked skin, sometimes followed by pain, inflammation, and swelling. Primarily found on the feet, the same fungus can infect other areas of the body, like the armpits, elbows, knees, and groin, which is why you guys should be careful putting on your undershorts. If they rub up against infected toes, your boxers or briefs may transfer the fungus to your crotch, resulting in jock itch, more formally known as *tinea cruris,* or "vermin of the crotch." (And, of course, never touch your genitals with your feet.)

To control athlete's foot, go barefoot as often as possible, wash feet frequently, dry your feet well after showering, and change socks daily. Topical fungicide ointments are very helpful.

One oddball therapy involves peeing on your feet. Proponents of urine therapy say that the natural urea found in pee is just like the urea found in topical ointments. Biochemists beg to differ, claiming the urea in the ointments is not antifungal, but just softens the skin to allow the fungicide to penetrate. (But what the heck, if you are going to pee in the shower anyway . . .)

What drug is made from the pee of old ladies?

Pergonal is a natural purified drug that is derived from the urine of postmenopausal women (old ladies). It has two hormones—follicle-stimulating hormone (FSH) and luteinizing hormone (LH)—that are gonadotropins, or sex hormones, that originate in the pituitary gland. The hormones in Pergonal can be used in fertility treatments to stimulate the ovaries to develop mature follicles that contain eggs. Pergonal is administered by intramuscular injections. It became available in the 1960s from the Italian company Serono. They set up urine-collection centers at convents throughout Italy, where they asked the elderly (postmenopausal) nuns for contributions. Because Pergonal was made from natural sources (old lady pee), it was quite pricey. Treatments averaged $1,400 a month in 1992. It was largely replaced by synthetic forms of urinary gonadotropins by 2000.

Many other drugs are made from urine or urea. Uro-kinase has human urine as an ingredient. It is used as a blood clot dissolver for unblocking clogged arteries (more on this later). Murine eardrops are made from carbamide peroxide. What is carbamide? It's synthetic urea and hydrogen peroxide. Ureaphil is a diuretic made from urea; urofollitropin, a urine-extract fertility drug; Ureacin, a urea cream for skin problems; Amino-Cerv, a urea cream for cervical treatments. Some cosmetics companies use urea as a moisturizer in their expensive creams and lotions.

What bestselling women's drug is made from horse pee?

If you are a menopausal woman you probably are familiar with Premarin. It is the number one selling pharmaceutical prescribed for hormone-replacement therapy to lessen the hot flashes, night sweats, and vaginal dryness that may accompany menopause. It is also indicated to eliminate the risk of osteoporosis and reduce the chance of heart disease in women over 50. Premarin comes in many forms (pills, creams, patches, injectables), and yes, as the name—which is a contraction of the words *pregnant mares' urine*—suggests, it is made from horse pee.

When women go through menopause, their levels of estrogen fall some 40 to 60 percent, which brings on the aforementioned symptoms. Premarin, and Premarin-containing products like Prempro, Premphase, and Prempak, all contain coagulated estrogen derived from pregnant mares' urine. If you need proof of this fact, simply break open a pill and smell it.

Premarin was the most prescribed drug in America from 1975 until 1999. As of 2003, 9 million American women were taking Premarin. Sales have recently slackened due to a big flap about the treatment of the horses used to obtain the urine. The mares are raised on big pregnant mares' urine (PMU) farms where the horses are tied up in a tiny stall for the 6 months of the year that they are pregnant so their urine can be collected. Most of the foals born are sold for slaughter after being fattened up. Any mares that are not easily impregnated meet the same fate.

Because of pressure from animal rights groups, the sale of Premarin drugs has dropped off somewhat, and newer synthetic PMU drugs are gaining favor.

Who makes pharmaceuticals from your excrement?

This one will knock your socks off. The pee you deposit in a Porta John is liquid gold, figuratively and literally. The

Porta John company gets an endless supply of human urine. Being smart businesspeople, the executives don't just dump it out somewhere. They are actively involved in "human-sourced protein production." Essentially what they are doing is mining gold in human waste.

In collaboration with Pharmaceuticals.org, Inc., they have a program to filter out useful pharmaceuticals from your urine. Presently, they supply purified urokinase (discussed earlier in the chapter) and crude monocyte colony-stimulating factor, kallikrein, epidermal growth factor, and human urinary albumin. They have thus far been able to retrieve 27 different useful compounds from human waste and are looking for ways to use them for profit. (Maybe they should pay you for your urine, not the other way round.)

Those clever Porta John people even have special little commodes for hospital patients to collect excrement from patients being treated with toxic oncology and other drugs. They can recover and recycle many expensive drugs for reuse and avoid having them enter the ecosystem through sewage systems.

When was urine taxed?

Believe it or not, urine was once taxed by the Romans. In the first century, Emperor Nero imposed a tax on the collection of pee. The plebes (common people) in Roman society pissed into pots that were dumped into cesspools. The fluid was collected from the cesspools and used for a number of chemical processes, including tanning and laundering (it was a source of ammonia to whiten clothes). Roman slaves removed the greasy lanolin from wool by tramping on it in tubs of human urine.

The tax was lifted for a few years, but levied again on all public restrooms by Nero's successor, Vespasian. Reportedly, when Vespasian's son Titus complained to him about the disgusting nature of the tax, he held up a gold coin and replied, *"Non olet!"* (It doesn't stink!) This phrase is still used in some countries to imply that all money is dirty, regardless of the source. Even in modern times Vespasian's name has been attached to public street urinals. In Paris, they called them *vespasiennes* and in Rome, *vespasiani*.

What culture stored their food in urine? (and other urine trivia)

- The Vikings are believed to have stored their perishable foods in barrels of pee. They rinsed the food before eating it.
- Men spend an average of 45 seconds to take a leak; women need 79 seconds. The average person (whoever that is) will pee some 9,200 gallons in his or her lifetime (depending on how much coffee and beer that person drinks).

- Urine remained in toothpastes well into the 1700s. Dentists knew that the ammonia in urine was a great cleaning agent. Ammonia can still be found in toothpastes today.
- The Allies used urine-soaked pads as gas masks during World War I.

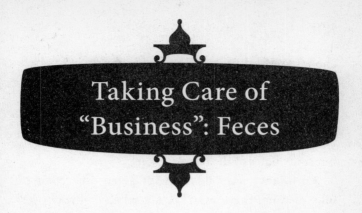

Taking Care of "Business": Feces

Unlike urine, fecal material is bacteria-laden and is definitely not good for you. However, some people (not just preteens) have a strange fascination with the stuff and are greatly amused by potty humor. Witness the popularity of the television show *South Park*. Although not everyone finds feces to be funny subject matter, even the most mature among you probably have a morbid curiosity about poop.

Why is poop brown?

The greatest proportion of your average turd is water. Water is removed from your fecal matter as it moves through the intestine, so the longer you retain it, the drier it will be. The next two largest components of feces are indigestible food, such as cellulose (also known as fiber) and dead bacteria from the intestines. There are also lesser amounts of live bacteria, dead cells, mucus, cholesterol, and inorganic salts. It's foul-smelling bacteria that make poop and farts stink (for more on farts, keep reading). Poop's brown coloration comes from bile and the pigment bilirubin, which comes from dead blood cells. The iron from blood hemoglobin in bilirubin contributes to the brown color.

An infant's feces is yellowish green—the color of bile—because they haven't produced any bilirubin yet. If a baby is breast-fed, the poop won't turn brown until the introduction of solid food.

Why are some bowel movements long and others little pieces?

Poop is usually one long, soft mass before it comes out of you. It often gets pinched into little pieces as you squeeze your sphincter muscles while defecating, kind of like what happens in a sausage-making machine. If you can keep your sphincter muscles relaxed, you may be able to produce a nice long log in the bowel. (Something to shoot for.)

Why does some poop float?

Because it's less dense than water. Some poop has a higher percentage of gas and thus floats. Other turds are high in fat content, causing them to bob along in the toilet.

Why does corn come out whole in your poop?

When you eat corn, it is unlikely that you chew up every last kernel. Usually some of the little guys are swallowed intact. It's these whole kernels that you will see speckled throughout your droppings shortly after eating corn. The reason whole kernels pass through you undigested is because their pericarp (outer layer) is made of cellulose, which the human digestive tract has not evolved to break down.

If corn poop bothers you, try chewing your corn kernels very thoroughly next time.

Why is diarrhea so watery?

The word *diarrhea* comes from the Greek word *diarrhein,* meaning "to flow through"—and that's exactly what diarrhea does in your body. When the intestines become irritated (from bacteria, viruses, strange food, and so on), they pass the food through your bowels very rapidly. This doesn't give the intestines time to remove much of the water from the fecal material and you get the squirts.

Can dietetic candy give you the runs?

If you eat sugar-free candies or put sugar-free syrup on your pancakes, chances are you are also ingesting sorbitol. It is a naturally occurring alcohol-based sweetener found in berries and some other fruits. Sorbitol is about half as sweet as sucrose (table sugar) and has the unique ability to retain moisture. For this reason, it is added to certain products to keep them moist and smooth. There is a drawback to this property, however. Ingesting too much sorbitol can give you diarrhea. Because it retains moisture in your bowels, it acts as a laxative.

An FDA warning, which reads "Excessive consumption may have a laxative effect" must appear on sorbitol-sweetened products. Other sugar substitutes in food are maltitol, mannitol, isomalt, xylitol, and hydrogenated starch hydrolysate. All of these additives can have a similar effect.

How do antidiarrheals work?

As mentioned earlier, diarrhea is caused by fecal material moving through the gut too fast. This doesn't give the intestines enough time to absorb moisture, so your poop comes out watery. Some antidiarrheals, such as Imodium, have an active ingredient called loperamide hydrochloride. Loperamide acts to slow the muscular contractions of the intestines (peristalsis) and so is termed an "antimotility" medicine. By acting on the opioid receptors found in the muscle lining of the intestinal walls, loperamide slows the movement of food and feces through the gut, allowing more time for the absorption of water and electrolytes into the body. The result is firmer, less frequent stools.

What foods can turn your poop bright green?

If the image of blue urine (discussed in the last chapter) amuses you, the thought of bright green poop should really make your day. Unlike colored urine, a green stool can easily be produced by eating too much of certain foods. A couple of kids' breakfast cereals will do the trick. Try Fruity Pebbles or Cap'n Crunch Berries, or Cap'n Crunch Swirled Berries. Purple Kool-Aid is also known to produce green berries, as it were, as will almost any drink containing blue dye. Even eating a cup of blueberries or lots of green leafy vegetables can result in a lovely kelly green log.

As every schoolchild knows, blue and yellow make green. This is what happens when you ingest enough blue dye. It mixes with your yellow bile and voilà—green poop! Most blue dyes don't turn your pee green because they don't get absorbed into the bloodstream and thus don't enter the kidneys.

You might have to drink several glasses of blue drinks or eat many bowls of cereal to obtain a lovely emerald specimen. Adolescent boys seem to really get a kick out of green poop, and for this reason are big consumers of blue Slurpees, grape soda, and Pepsi Blue. Ah, life's simple pleasures.

Other interesting stool colors can be achieved. Should you wish to produce black, iron supplements, Pepto-Bismol, or black licorice might do the trick. Beets, tomato soup or juice, and strawberry Jell-O can reward you with red droppings.

If you haven't been consuming large amounts of any of these foods and you have a crazy colored stool, it may indicate a medical problem for which you might want to consult a physician.

What is constipation?

OK, you all know what constipation is, but because it's pretty gross in some respects, we'll dwell on it for a short time. In quick review, constipation is the production of hard feces that are difficult to evacuate. Straining to void may cause hemorrhoids and anal tears.

Everyone's bowel movement routine is unique. Some folks go every day like clockwork. Others go as seldom as once a week. (Talk about a log.) Doctors have to take this into account when diagnosing constipation. Generally, if your turds are difficult to pass, are very hard, or are rabbit-like pellets, you are considered to be constipated, regardless of how frequently you go. Abdominal pain and bloating are also indicators.

Constipation can occur as a result of insufficient ingestion of fluids and fibers or from medication side effects. A doctor may be able to feel lumps of feces when he or she presses on your abdomen. A rectal exam will show whether or not there is poop in your lower rectum. Oral medicines, suppositories, or enemas may be indicated. Usually, increasing fibers and fluids is sufficient. In severe cases, manual extraction can be performed, after a sedative or general anesthetic is administered to loosen the sphincter.

Can constipation kill you?

Perhaps you have heard, a disproportionate number of people die while sitting on the toilet, considering the short amount of time they spend there. Statistics show that it is usually older men who are at higher risk.[1] Because they die while sitting down, you know what type of "business" these guys were conducting when they met their end, as it were. But why? Maybe you could guess the answer if you knew that most of them suffer heart attacks while defecating. Yes, it's the deadly combination of weak heart and constipation.

Constipated older men and women push harder and longer while on the toilet, doing what is called a Valsalva maneuver—forcibly exhaling with closed lips and nostrils (bet you didn't know this toilet technique had a fancy name). This puts pressure on the intestines and colon and creates additional pressure on the abdominal and thoracic (chest) cavities. The major veins leading back to the heart are usually held open by lower pressure in the chest cavity around these vessels. An increase in thoracic pressure can pinch the vessels off, preventing blood from flowing back to the heart. When receptors in the heart detect a significant drop in pressure, they cause a pressure spike—which can lead to a heart attack.

Why do you often need to defecate after eating?

In a word—peristalsis. This is the squeezing action of the intestines that moves food and digested waste through the gastrointestinal tract. Eating stimulates peristalsis, pushing everything along toward the anus.

What are the seven different types of poop?

You didn't know that there are seven types of poop, did you? There is a chart that doctors use to determine the kind of bowel movements that their patients are trying to describe to them. Known as the Bristol Stool Chart, it was developed at the University of Bristol, in England, by K. W. Heaton, in 1990.[2]

Before the chart was created, doctors had to ask patients to describe their poop as graphically as possible. This was not only somewhat less than accurate, it also could be rather embarrassing. Now, with the stool chart, patients can simply point out the shape and texture of their movements with a greater degree of accuracy and a little less embarrassment.

The Bristol Stool Chart defines seven stool types, arranged by shape and consistency, with a color (guess which one) picture of each turd type:

- *Type 1:* Separate hard lumps, like nuts, hard to pass
- *Type 2:* Sausage-shaped, but lumpy

- *Type 3:* Like a sausage, but with cracks on its surface
- *Type 4:* Like sausage or snake, smooth and soft
- *Type 5:* Soft blobs with clear-cut edges, easily passed
- *Type 6:* Fluffy pieces with ragged edges, a mushy stool
- *Type 7:* Watery, no solid pieces, entirely liquid

As mentioned earlier, the form of your stool depends on how long it spent in the colon. Types 1 and 2 indicate constipation. Types 3 and 4 are the most comfortable to pass. Types 5 and 6 tend to pass with urgency. Type 7 is diarrhea.

If you are curious as to the type of stool you are passing, there's no need to see a doctor. Just go online and type "Bristol Stool Chart" into your search engine. Then compare your findings with friends.

What popular fragrance and flavoring is now made from cow dung?

The chemical vanillin is responsible for giving the vanilla bean its wonderful aroma and flavor. Artificial vanillin is much cheaper than that extracted from vanilla beans. Synthetic vanillin was patented by a German chemist in 1875. It is identical to natural vanillin and can be found in imitation vanilla extract. From 1875 to 1925, vanillin was made from clove oils. From 1925 until the present, it has been made from paper industry wood-pulp by-products (lignin). But that is changing.

Japanese researchers have succeeded in making the sweet smell of vanilla from one of the most offensive-smelling things around—cow dung. Through a 1-hour heating and pressurizing process, cow droppings will produce vanillin. Chemically, it's identical to vanillin from vanilla beans, and its cost is one-half that of the original's. Its creators foresee its use in shampoos and candles, but not in food, as most people would not be willing to accept it.

Why would anyone do such research? you may ask. Well, there's a lot of cow pies in the world and more are on the way. A main component of dung is lignin from the grass the cows eat. It is very difficult to decompose, and farmers are at a loss as to how to get rid of it. Enter the researchers. After taking the vanillin from the lignin, the recycled poop can be returned to the soil.

Why is bird poop white?

Because of uric acid. Unlike us, birds don't urinate. Our kidneys remove nitrogenous wastes from the blood and excrete it in the form of urea dissolved in our pee. Birds excrete it as uric acid, which is a not very soluble combination of poop and pee. If you ever take a hard look at that white plop on your windshield, you will notice that the center of the dropping is a soft mass. This is the poo. That watery slime around the edge is the pee.

Bird poop is released from the cloaca—a multi-use orifice that also is used for egg laying and sex. All birds, amphibians, and reptiles have a cloaca. Why bird droppings have an uncanny knack for landing on just-washed cars is still one of life's great mysteries.

How was dog poop used to make leather?

Tanneries in ancient times were such a disgusting business that they were allowed only on the outskirts of towns. They smelled something terrible.

Skins arrived at a tanner's dried out, stiff as a board, and caked with guts. The first thing tanners did was soften a hide by soaking it in water. Next, the bits of flesh and blood were removed by pounding and scouring. To remove hairs from the hide, the tanners would coat them with an alkaline lime mixture, soak them in urine, or let them sit out for months to putrefy, before being scraped.

The process gets even grosser. Bating, which further softened the skins, was next. Tanners pounded or kneading the skins in a watery solution of dog or pigeon poop. The kneading would take several hours and was done by hand or by the tanner walking on the hides in bare feet. Skins could also be made more supple by soaking them in a slurry of puréed animal brains.

Children in the towns were employed to gather

animal droppings, and washerwomen would collect urine from pots left out on street corners.

Any leftover bits of leather were turned into glue by being left in vats of water to deteriorate for several months. This mushy mess was then boiled off to yield hide glue.

Why do farts stink?

The gas that comes out of your back end is made up of many different things: swallowed air, gas made by bacteria in the gut, gas from chemical reactions in the gut, and blood gases seeping into the digestive tract. At any one time, there is a different mix of these gases and foods present in your gastrointestinal tract, meaning the smell of your farts will vary.

The air you swallow is absorbed by the body on its way through the gastrointestinal tract. When it reaches the large intestine, it is mainly nitrogen. Carbon dioxide may also be found there, formed by chemical interactions between stomach acids and intestinal fluids.

Hydrogen and methane are generated by bacterial action. Farts contain low levels of other gases, such as hydrogen sulfide and mercaptans (other sulfur-containing organic chemicals) as well as nitrogen compounds like indole and skatole—all of which reek. These same chemicals make poop stink. Foods containing sulfur will contribute to smellier farts. Cauliflower, eggs, and meat can increase the stink factor, whereas beans will lead to more prodigious, but less smelly gas.

Why are "silent-but-deadly" farts so nasty?

You all know what these nasty guys are! Your common everyday fart is largely nitrogen and carbon dioxide from swallowed air. They are usually big gas bubbles that leave the anus at normal body temperature and can produce a nice acoustic effect and may or may not pack a wallop. The silent-but-deadly fart is a different animal altogether—a very smelly one. These guys are the byproduct of bacterial activity. Bacterial fermentation and digestion generate some wicked-smelling gases and heat, creating those silent-but-deadly farts. As you are aware, they can be rather hot, and small, allowing them to slip out quietly, without causing the sphincter muscles to vibrate. They may, however, cause a decided reaction from any innocent bystanders in the vicinity.

Why do beans make you fart?

Some people are more susceptible to bean gas than others. The problem with legumes, especially beans, is their high fiber and oligosaccharide (complex sugar) content. The human digestive tract lacks the enzymes required to break down these sugars. In beans, the offending sugar is called raffinose. Lima and navy beans are the worst culprits in the legume family. High levels of oligosaccharides are also found in some of the other major gas-producing foods—broccoli, Brussels sprouts, cabbage, and cauliflower.

Because these complex sugars are not broken down in the upper intestine, they travel to the lower intestine whole, where bacteria begin working on them. As discussed, bacterial action releases some noxious gases. In a way, this bean intolerance is analogous to lactose intolerance, wherein a person doesn't have the enzymes needed to digest dairy products, resulting in bacterial fermentation and gas.

How can you fart less?

Aside from just holding them in, which *is* an option, there are less painful ways. Some people who eat a lot of gas-producing foods seem to build up a tolerance for them. Gradually increasing your intake could help. Other lifestyle changes you could make (if you are *really* averse to farting) would be to restrict gas-producing activities—chewing gum, drinking or eating too fast, and drinking soda—all of which cause you to swallow air, adding to your gassiness.

Over-the-counter remedies are also available. If your flatulence is a problem for you, try Beano. It contains the missing enzyme—beta-galactosidase—which is necessary for the bacteria to do their work. Just take Beano next time you eat beans and you should be fine.

Another pill on the market is Flatulex. It takes a different approach to the problem. Flatulex contains activated carbon to absorb some of the odors while they are still in you.

Does flying give you gas?

The decreased cabin pressure at altitude may increase your gas woes and the woes of your fellow passengers. You may think this is funny, but don't laugh. During World War II, the U.S. government conducted studies to determine the effect of flatulence on high-altitude pilots. NASA later did likewise.

As you may or may not remember from your high school physics class, the volume of a gas increases as the pressure around it decreases. In an unpressurized cabin this could cause the flight crew some small discomfort. It was even thought that too much intestinal gas in an enclosed cockpit would prove detrimental to the pilots. We're thankful that the gas pressure is easily released.

Why do farts burn after eating spicy food?

If you are a fan of real spicy food, you have probably experienced this annoying phenomenon. Why? The oils in these foods are not digested, but pass all the way through your gastrointestinal tract intact, burning on the way out.

Can you light a fart on fire?

What 12-year-old boy hasn't pondered this age-old question or even conducted his own test? Well, yes, Virginia (or Johnny), you can indeed light a fart on fire. In fact, the practice is so common that it goes by several different names, including blue angel, blue blazer, blue dart, and blue flame.

As mentioned earlier, a fart contains gases like methane and hydrogen (remember the *Hindenburg*?), which are very flammable. Blue flames come from farts containing methane. Only about one-third of the population is believed to have methane farts. (Who studies this stuff?) However, orange and yellow flames may also be produced, depending on the particular blend of gases and bacteria emitted by your colon at any particular time.

For legal reasons we will not go into detail on the best ways to light your farts, but suffice it to say you should be ***very careful***, as the potential to burn your privates is rather high. (Remember, if you suffer personal injury, you didn't get the fart-lighting idea here.)

While you may think this is funny, take heed. There are documented cases of bodily gases igniting in operating rooms. Electric sparks during colon (or more rarely abdominal) surgery can result in an explosion of trapped methane gas![3] (Very gross.) This can lead to serious injury or death of the patient. Nursing professionals recommend putting a wet sponge into the rectum during procedures on or near the anal area while using an electrosurgical unit or laser.[4]

Why do dog farts smell so bad?

Did you ever hear a dog fart? How about a cat? No? This is because they are carnivores and eat a lot of protein-rich meat. As noted earlier, high-protein diets result in highly pungent gas, delivered in low doses. Add to this the fact that many pet foods contain soybean meal (beans!) and that animal's sphincters are not as tight as our own, and you can see why dogs and cats deliver silent-but-really-deadly farts.

Is it dangerous to hold in a fart? (and other fart trivia)

- The medical term for farting is *flatulence,* which comes from the Latin *flatus,* which means "the act of blowing."
- People fart the most upon rising from bed. This is known as "morning thunder."
- It is not harmful to hold in a fart. People who do simply let them rip in their sleep.
- Emperor Claudius once passed a law making it legal to fart at banquets. He thought holding them in could poison you.

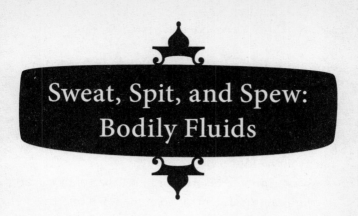

Sweat, Spit, and Spew: Bodily Fluids

A lot of foul-smelling and -tasting fluids are found within our bodies. The more repulsive ones are those that commonly exit the body—sweat, saliva, and vomit. Different people have different thresholds of disgust when it comes to bodily fluids. Obviously, doctors, nurses, and veterinarians have a higher level of disgust than the average Joe. Even they, however, do not relish sweat, spit, and spew.

Why does puke taste so foul?

Contrary to popular myth, vomit does not taste bad from your stomach acids. These actually have no taste, although they will cause a burning sensation in your mouth. Three other culprits are responsible for the bad taste of barf.

The unforgettable smell and taste of puke comes from butyl acid, which is brought up from the depths of your small intestine. Also, all kinds of digested and partly digested foods all mixed together can taste pretty funky, too. Finally, there are no sweets in vomit. Sugars are the first things to be broken down in the digestive process. They start to be broken down as soon as they enter your mouth.

About 1 minute before you puke, the vomit center in your brain sends a message to the small intestine to send a good portion of its contents back into the stomach. This helps neutralize the highly corrosive stomach acids in the vomit, making it less damaging to the esophagus, throat, mouth, and teeth. It is also likely that the toxins your body is rejecting were first detected in the small intestine, so purging it is essential. In addition, the transfer of intestinal matter into the stomach increases its contents, making vomiting easier. You see, the more stuff in your stomach, the easier it will be to puke a second or third time, if necessary. An empty stomach will lead to the dreaded dry heaves.

Why is vomiting contagious?

Did you ever feel like puking when in close proximity to someone else who is? How about just catching a whiff of fresh, warm vomit? It almost makes you gag just thinking about it, kind of like wanting to yawn when someone else does, only much grosser. It has been suggested that this reaction is an evolved behavior in primates. Wild primates tend to forage together and eat the same foods. If one member of the group becomes ill, it probably isn't a bad evolutionary strategy for the others to throw up right away, in case they are all eating something bad.

One indicator as to how fundamentally repulsive we all find puking is the results of a survey to determine the worst sound in the world.[1] The study was conducted by Trevor Cox of the University of Salford's Accoustic Research Centre, in England. He set up a project called BadVibes, with 34 sounds for online test subjects to rate. After 1 year and 1.1 million votes, the sound of someone vomiting was chosen as the most disgusting. The sound was re-created by an actor using a diluted bucket of baked beans to simulate puke cascading into a toilet. Lovely.

What causes projectile vomiting?

If regular puking is gross, projectile vomiting is off-the-charts gross. You know what this is. It happens to kids way more than to adults. Instead of starting to feel nauseous, retching a little, and bending over to barf, you just spew the entire contents of your stomach straight out across the room. During a projectile event, the throat closes to a little hole that the vomit must pass through. Just like when you put your thumb over the end of a garden hose to make it squirt farther, the same thing happens to your barf here. Look out!

A recent study of puking in restaurants found that anyone in the same room as a vomiter may get infected with the germs spewed out. People at the same table were most likely to get sick, but folks at tables some distance from the puker were also at risk.[2] The study concluded that restaurants need to disinfect much larger areas than most do when cleaning up barf.

Who pukes more, men or women?

Can you guess this one? Yes, it's women. One recent barfing survey (don't ask) found that on average, women vomit 5 times a year compared to 1.5 times for men.[3] One reason for this may be that women find being nauseous more unbearable than do men. Morning sickness during pregnancy may also skew the results.

Want some more vomiting trivia?

- People in Europe vomit more than Americans, who vomit more than Canadians. Americans in the north vomit more than folks in the south.
- For banquets, ancient Romans had special rooms called *vomitoriums,* where stuffed dinner guests would go to upchuck and make room for more food.

Why do you start to salivate just before puking?

You all know that feeling. Whether you had a long night of drinking or are just coming down with a 24-hour virus, it's unmistakable. Your stomach begins to feel uneasy and your mouth starts to water—in a bad way. What's the purpose of this saliva?

Vomit contains gastric juices from the stomach. These are very corrosive and can erode your tooth enamel. The teeth need protection. As you prepare to puke, your brain sends signals to your salivary glands to get busy. Then when you barf, the slightly alkaline saliva is already there to help neutralize the acids and form a protective coating on your teeth.

Where do people spit on newborns to bring the child good luck?

Spit grosses out a lot of people, but it really is amazing stuff. You salivate all the time. Your salivary glands, found inside each cheek and under the tongue, squirt out between 2 and 4 cups of spit every day. You couldn't swallow, kiss, or talk without it. Thick and colorless, spit is constantly bathing your mouth. As you can guess, it's mainly made up of water (95 percent) with some other goodies mixed in, like electrolytes, mucus, proteins, mineral salts, antibacterial compounds, and enzymes.

One enzyme in saliva begins the process of digestion even before the food makes it to the stomach. Saliva also has high concentrations of calcium and phosphate ions, the materials teeth are made of. When microscopic lesions occur in the tooth enamel, these ions can remineralize them.

That's the good stuff. Spit also has numerous kinds of bacteria, viruses, and fungi, which find the warm, dark, wet environment to their liking. Leftover bits of food have plenty of places to hide in the mouth and are always there for microbes to feast on. Despite all the bacteria in your mouth, you will very rarely get an infection when you bite the inside of your lip, cheek, or tongue. This is because in addition to bacteria, spit has plenty of antibiotics and antimicrobial compounds. This is one reason people are much less likely to become infected with HIV from oral sex than from other types of sexual contact. Proteins in saliva that promote the formation of blood vessels help wounds in the mouth heal quicker than wounds on the skin, and without scarring.

Finally, saliva helps the body regulate its water levels because a lack of it stimulates the sensation of thirst.

Yes, spit is a marvelous thing. It seems to gross out a lot of folks, but not the Masai people of Tanzania. They consider it a show of goodwill. Traders seal deals by spitting on one another, and newborn babies are spat on to bring the child good luck (and maybe a few germs).

Is it good to lick your wounds?

As we have seen, spit has good bacteria and bad bacteria. It also has proteins, antibiotics, and antimicrobials. So is it helpful to lick your wounds, like a dog? Research on this subject has been, to date, inconclusive. Licking your wounds might not be a bad idea, if you can't get to soap and water quickly. Licking will clean the wound of any large contaminants, such as dirt, and may brush away some infective agents.

Why don't kids stink when they sweat?

Your body is capable of losing several quarts of perspiration during vigorous activity. This is how you stay cool. A pea-size drop of sweat can cool about 1 quart of blood about 1°F. Happily, only around 1 percent of your body's perspiration is produced under the arms; it just feels like more.

Perhaps you didn't know, but there are two types of sweat glands: eccrine and apocrine. You are born with eccrine sweat glands. They are the most numerous and are especially abundant on the palms of the hands, soles of the feet, and the forehead. Eccrine sweat glands produce mainly water and salt and are key in body temperature regulation.

The apocrine glands are found in areas of abundant hair follicles, like the underarms and genitals. They don't begin to function until after the onset of puberty. Apocrine glands are the main cause of body odor, due to the bacterial breakdown of the organic fatty compounds they secrete. Because children don't have these glands, they don't have much body odor (at least not from sweating, anyway). Something else you may not have known: Breasts are a modified form of the apocrine sweat gland.

Sweat glands are found in the middle layer of the skin—the dermis. They are long, coiled tubes of cells. The sweat is made in the bottom, coiled part and is secreted through a long, straight neck that extends up to a pore at the surface of the skin.

One last bit of sweat trivia—the only areas of skin on the body that do not sweat are the nail bed, the margins of the lips, the eardrums, and the tip of the penis.

Why do some people's feet smell like cheese?

The Dutch have a word for foot odor—*tenenkaas*—or "toe cheese" (not to be confused with Cheetos). The only real thing feet have in common with cheese is bacteria, and that's the answer to the question. Cheese is made through the controlled "spoilage" of milk. In the process lactose, proteins, and milk fats are broken down into some rather odoriferous by-products. The same by-products are given off by the microbes that live in the dank, dark places on your body, especially the feet.

Under the right conditions, bacteria can really have a feast on your feet. They love dead skin cells and oils from your skin. If you don't wear socks, your foot moisture will cause bacteria to take up residence in your shoes, making them reek.

If you have ever smelled Limburger cheese, it may have reminded you of really stinky feet. That's because Limburger is made using the bacterium *Brevibacterium linens,* which is very closely related to the stinky feet bacterium *Brevibacterium epidermis.* About 38 percent of people have feet that harbor *B. epidermis.* Those that have it, have plenty of it—something like a million bacteria on the web between each toe. *B. epidermis*'s partner in smelliness is the bacterium *Micrococcus sedentarius.*

So how did the same bacterium that causes foot odor get into Limburger cheese? Simple. The Trappist monks of Limburg, Belgium, who first created the cheese in the eighteenth century, would mix the curds and milk into cheese by stomping it with their feet. So, in essence, when you eat Limburger, you are eating the same bacterium found in toe jam. Yummy!

But even feet that aren't home to stinky bacteria smell. This is because of fatty acids from the breakdown of fat substances in degenerating skin cells.

If cheese smells like stinky feet, why do we like cheese?

There are some folks who have an aversion to the smell of cheese. Deep in our primordial brain, we are hard-wired to be disgusted by the smell of spoiled food. When humans started intentionally spoiling (fermenting) foods, we had to overcome this revulsion. The attraction for fragrant cheeses is thus an acquired one. Some people never overcome this revulsion.

Why do some people's feet *really* stink?

There's a medical term for *really* smelly feet— bromidrosis. Between 10 and 20 percent of people have extra-smelly feet. This is because they have extra-sweaty feet, which become home to the bacterium *M. sedentarius*. These bacteria not only produce the normal smelly by-products mentioned earlier but also release more noxious volatile sulfur compounds (VSCs), which smell of rotten eggs.

When did athletes sell their sweat?

The ancient Romans and Greeks didn't use soap to wash. Instead, they coated their bodies with perfumed oils and then scraped them off with a curved metal tool called a strigil. People of means had their slaves do this for them. The oily mess scraped away contained their dirt, sweat, and dead skin cells. During the Greek Olympics, athletes would oil up before competing and be scraped down with a strigil afterward. The star athletes would put their disgusting scrapings in little bottles and sell them to younger, aspiring athletes who hoped they might confer on them some of their former owner's athletic abilities.

What is eye sand?

Also called sleepers (sleep, sleepies), eye crust, and eye gunk, this is the crud you get in your eyes when you sleep. Did you ever notice those little bumps of red tissue in the corners of your eyes closest to your nose? They are called the caruncles (everything has a name, doesn't it?). Your caruncles are lumps of flesh that are composed of oil and sweat glands. They squirt out the white crud that sometimes collects in the corner of your eye, but these bumps aren't the only source of eye crust.

Each eye has about 30 glands that create tears that bathe and cleanse the eyeball. In a year's time, over 8 pints of tears will have flowed across your eyeballs and either evaporated or drained away in the corner of your eye. These old tears flow down into your throat, where you swallow them. This is why your nose runs when you cry.

When you sleep, your eyelids are screwed tight. The few night tears that you make pool in the corner of your eye because the little drain holes close when your eyes are shut. When the stuff in your tears dries out and mixes with the oil and sweat from your caruncles, you get eye crud. The sleepers in your eyelashes are tears that have seeped out between your eyelids and evaporated, leaving behind a little crust.

How much snot do you make in a day?

Snot is basically mucus that is produced to protect the lungs. Mucus, like most bodily fluids, is mostly water, 95 percent in fact. The rest is salt and mucin, a sticky protein that is used in some animal-based glues. The air you breathe is full of particles like dust, dirt, pollen, and germs. If this stuff made it all the way to your lungs, they could become irritated or infected, making it tough to breathe. The moist, sticky mucus in your nose traps most of these things. Small hairs in your nose, called cilia, help move your dirty, germy snot to the back of the throat. Each hair sweeps 10 times a second, moving the snot along at the brisk pace of ¼ inch a minute. When the traveling snot reaches the back of your throat, you unconsciously swallow most of it. How much do you swallow? The average healthy person makes about a cupful of snot every day. To keep up with demand, your nose makes a new batch of mucus every 20 minutes.

As the mucus dries out, you get boogers—the stuff many are fond of picking. The production of boogers is a sign of a normally functioning nose.

A "loogie" is vernacular for a mass of phlegm spit from the throat of someone with nasal congestion. Its name probably derives from a combination of the words *lunger,* the expectoration (spit) of a person with tuberculosis, and *booger.*

A "snot rocket," if you don't know, is the mucoid projectile that you can shoot out of one nostril while holding shut the opposing nostril. This is an option for those without a tissue or sleeve to blow into.

Babies don't know how to blow the snot out of their nose. Modern mothers use little rubber suction bulbs to suck out the snot. Eskimo mothers traditionally sucked out baby's snot with their mouths and spat it on the ground.

During the Middle Ages, it was acceptable to pick your nose in polite company. Etiquette books of the time advised that one scoop out boogers with one finger, as opposed to two, so as not to appear rude. Whether it was to be flicked or eaten is less clear.

Why does your nose run in cold weather?

Even if you are perfectly healthy, your nose will run when you are outside for a while on a cold day. This is because the cilia that are supposed to sweep the mucus to the back of your throat slow down or stop moving altogether when it's real cold. So the mucus just drips out of your nose. Mucus also thickens when exposed to cold temperatures. This is why your nose may run worse upon going inside to warm up. The mucus thaws and begins to drip before the cilia start working again.

Why is snot green?

Actually, it's not. Snot is crystal clear when it is made. After it picks up junk from the air it becomes opaque. That grody yellow-green snot that clogs you up when you have a cold gets its funky color from bacteria and bacterial wastes.

Is your earwax brown or gray?

The ears collect a lot of crud. We all get wax in our ears. But what is this stuff? Earwax, or cerumen, isn't really wax, not paraffin (candle wax) anyway. It is a sticky liquid that is secreted by sebaceous glands, and modified apocrine sweat glands found only in the skin of the ear canals. These glands are related to the apocrine glands found in the armpits and breasts.

One function of earwax is to keep your ear canal moist and viscous. It also inhibits bacteria and fungal growth there. Being sticky, earwax traps all kinds of junk that enters your ear. Everything from, dirt, sweat, and oil, to bugs, bacteria, and bits of plant material get stuck in this stuff. Its primary function is to keep all this junk out of your ear canal and eardrum.

You may not have known this, but there are two types of earwax—wet and dry. Most white people of European descent and African Americans have the wet type, which is brown and moist. About 85 percent of white American women have wet earwax, while virtually all African Americans do. Most East Asians have the dry variety, which is gray and flaky. Intermediate frequencies (30 to 50 percent) of the dry type are seen in populations of southern Asia, the Pacific Islands, central Asia, and Asia Minor, as well as people of native North American and Asian Inuit ancestry.

Although everybody has earwax, some folks never have to clean it out of their ears. It just doesn't accumulate. As new wax forms, it pushes forward the old wax, which falls out in tiny clumps or flakes as they move their jaws. If you have too much earwax it can affect your hearing. Some people with very hard earwax can feel discomfort from pressure on the sensitive ear canal walls. Because the ear canal shares some nerves with the throat, an earwax buildup can cause a tickling sensation there and lead to a cough.

Do you have bugs in your ears?

You'd be surprised how many emergency room visits there are for people who get bugs in their ears. One common uninvited ear visitor is the cockroach, who enjoys crawling into small, dark places. Spiders have been known to live in children's ears. Japanese beetles have even been reported to chew right through the eardrum! Emergency room doctors know exactly what to do to evict these unwanted guests. They pour oil into the ear to drown the pest, then pull it out with tweezers.

How is a candle used to remove earwax?

People get all kinds of things stuck in their ears and often damage their eardrums in the process. The old adage "Never put anything in your ear smaller than your elbow" came about for good reason. Yet, most people ignore this sage advice and use Q-tips or some such implement to extract their wax. Cotton swabs are fine if you are very careful and don't probe too deeply. If you have a severe wax problem, they will do more harm than good, forcing the wax farther into the ear canal. Some people actually have wax plugs that can be an inch long!

What's the proper way to clean out your ears? Doctors irrigate the ears by squirting warm water into the ear canal to rinse the goop out. Failing that, they will scoop it out with a curette (a small tool with a metal ring at the end) or remove it by suction.

One home remedy gaining in popularity is "candling," or "coning." One end of a hollowed-out candle is placed in the ear canal, while the wick at the other end is lit, allowing it to burn for a short time. Supposedly, the burning flame creates a vacuum at the other end, sucking out all the nasty crud inside. When the candle is removed, the end will appear dark brown, indicating that the wax has been removed. Healthcare professionals warn against such a foolish practice, saying that it is ineffective and may result in ear burns or infections.

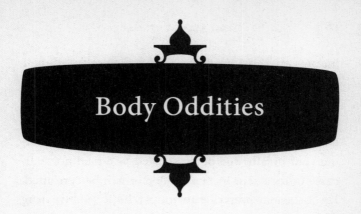

Body Oddities

The human body is a beautiful thing, but at times it can be totally gross. There is a multitude of disgusting conditions that those of you not in the medical field may be repulsed by. Speaking of the medical profession (is there any grosser field of endeavor?), there are also loads of medical procedures and techniques that will make your skin crawl, if you really think about them. Well, here's your chance.

Can a rectal exam cure the hiccups?

You may have tried any number of odd remedies to cure a bout of hiccups, but it's unlikely that you tried this one! Hiccups are a repeated involuntary spasm of the diaphragm. A sudden rush of air into the lungs causes the glottis (the space between the vocal cords) to close, making the familiar *hic* sound. Most bouts with hiccups are short-lived and resolve themselves of their own accord.

There are many folk remedies for stopping hiccups, including drinking a glass of water while holding one's nose, swallowing a teaspoon of sugar and holding your breath, and being startled by a loud noise. In cases of incessant hiccups, a doctor can be consulted. He or she may prescribe an antipsychotic sedative drug such as Haldol or Thorazine or a gastrointestinal stimulant such as Reglan. Antispasmodic drugs may also be helpful.

One cure you may not be familiar with involves, of all things, the rectum! In 2006, Francis Fesmire of the University of Tennessee College of Medicine received an Ig Nobel Prize in medicine for his 1988 paper titled "Termination of Intractable Hiccups with Digital Rectal Massage."[1] Yes, it's just what you think it is. By sticking his finger into someone's anus and massaging the rectum, he was able to cure a bout of severe, long-term hiccups. By stimulating the vagus nerve (part of the system of nerves that controls the movement of the bowels and the heart rate), he found that he could interrupt the nerve signals that were causing the contractions of the diaphragm. According to Fesmire, one curious side effect of "incredible" stimulation of the vagus nerve is an orgasm. There are, however, less invasive ways to stimulate the vagus, such as massaging a carotid artery or pulling on the earlobes. But these techniques may not be as effective.

The world's record for longest bout of the hiccups belongs to Charles Osborne (1894–1991) of Anthon,

Iowa, who hiccupped continuously from 1922 to 1990, a total of 68 years.[2] (Guess he never had his rectum digitally massaged.)

Where are skin-eating fish used in psoriasis therapy?

Here's another one from the incredible-but-true file. Psoriasis is a chronic disease that causes red scaly patches of skin. An excess of skin cell production results in an accumulation of skin in the affected areas. There are many different treatment options, but none is surefire. The treatment that is the most unusual, and claimed to be the best by its adherents, is given by the so-called fishy spas of Kangal, Turkey.

These indoor and outdoor spas are pools formed from the water of hot springs. The pools' temperatures approach 95°F. They are stocked with two species of carp-like fish from the Tigris and Euphrates Rivers: *Cyprinion macrostomus* and *Garra rufa*, also known as "strikers" and "lickers." The fish range in size from 6 to 8 inches. The spa's owners refer to them collectively as "doctor fish," because of what they do.

Psoriasis patients go to these spas and sit in the pools of fishy water for 4 hours at a time, twice a day. The doctor fish have no other source of food available, so they nibble on the patients' flaky skin cells that have been softened up by the hot water! The strikers feed more aggressively than the lickers, hence their respective names. The bather is said to at first experience a pleasant "micro-massage" sensation, followed by a tingling feeling all over the skin.

After about 3 weeks, the fish will have eaten off all the scales, causing minor bleeding, and exposing the lesions to sunlight and the water. The ultraviolet sunlight at these high-altitude spas and the presence of selenium in their waters is very therapeutic.

You can buy doctor fish from dealers in Germany and do your own at-home treatment, if you're so inclined.

Can a human ear grow on the back of a mouse?

Try to imagine a fully formed human ear growing on the back of a naked mouse. This may sound like some bizarro creation from a bad sci-fi movie, but it's a medical reality brought to us by the wonders of modern technology. Scientists can now grow a full-size human ear on the back of a mouse! Charles Vacanti, a transplant surgeon at Massachusetts General Hospital in Boston, did just this in 1997.

Vacanti used a frame made of biodegradable plastic mesh shaped like an ear. The frame was dipped into a solution of cartilage cells and then in a nutrient solution. The cells multiplied and linked together. The mold was attached under the skin on the back of a hairless mouse, where it was fed from the mouse's blood. When the frame dissolved, the result was a full-size human ear ready for transplant. The same technique has also been used to create noses.

You can go online and view the incredibly bizarre photos of these mice. Type "ear mouse" into your browser and get ready for a severe case of the willies!

What should you do if you cut off your finger (God forbid)?

First thing, don't panic. You probably have 12 hours to get it sewn back on (so you can finish cutting the firewood first, if you wish). If you put your finger in the refrigerator, you can wait a couple of days, although the blood gushing out of the stump on your hand may preclude this.

But, seriously, what should you do with a displaced piece of your body? Well, doctors highly recommend sealing it in a plastic bag and putting it on ice. Don't place it directly on ice, as this may cause frostbite (you don't need that problem on top of the one you already have!). Placing your severed body part in water will make it harder to reattach.

Some detached body parts may require more immediate attention than others. Fingers and penises are pretty durable on their own for a while. (Remember John Wayne Bobbitt?) Also, any parts that are mainly made of cartilage, like the ears and nose, have a slow metabolism and can be stored for several days. Body parts with more muscle tissue and a faster rate of metabolism are a little more perishable. Arms or legs should be sewn back on in 6 to 12 hours, tops.

How do they reattach body parts?

Say you've got a stray body part and have packed it in ice—how is it reattached to you? Restoring blood flow is key. You have to hope that the part has arteries large enough to be manipulated through microsurgery. Generally speaking, this means 1.5 millimeters or larger in diameter. The arteries bring new blood into the piece. The veins, which carry the blood back out, must also be reattached. If the veins cannot be sewn back together right away, leeches can be placed on the body part to reduce swelling. (More on leeches in a minute.) Bones, tendons, and nerves also need to be reattached. Things like ears that don't really have big arteries to work with are a little dicey. A clean cut, of course, makes the surgeons' job much easier.

How were leeches used by doctors?

Leeches recall the dark ages of medicine, when doctors did more harm than good. For centuries they were the mainstay of European medical practice. The word *leech* even comes from the Old English word *laece,* meaning "physician."

Ever since the time of Hippocrates, who believed disease was caused by an imbalance of the body's four humors—blood, black bile (poop), yellow bile (vomit), and phlegm (mucus)—doctors have been practicing bloodletting to restore the proper balance. The Greeks believed too much of any humor made you sick: Too much black bile gave you diarrhea, too much yellow bile made you barf, and too much phlegm gave you a cold. Because poop, puke, and mucus naturally come out of the body, the removal of some blood was needed to keep everything in balance.

Leeches (*Hirudo medicinalis*) were used for local bloodletting to reduce swelling and inflammation. They are particularly good for removing excess blood from areas of the body that other tools cannot reach, such as the cervix, hemorrhoids, and tonsils. To attach them to such tricky areas, doctors used glass tubes through which the slimy creatures would crawl to the target area. It wasn't until the early twentieth century, when medical research showed they were ineffective for most diseases, that leeches fell out of favor.

Do medicinal leeches ever wander into body orifices?

By the 1980s, leeches were back. Plastic surgeons rediscovered their ability to relieve venous congestion in grafts and transplants: A leech is left in place for 30 to 60 minutes, after which time it falls off, having removed about 20 milliliters of blood. Fresh leeches may be applied for days or weeks, until the congestion is relieved and the veins begin to drain the blood normally. And after they are finished sucking the blood, they can be eaten. (Just kidding!)

In the old days, people gathered leeches by wading into infested waters and letting them attach to their legs. "Leech catcher" was an actual paid job in Europe. Leeches are commercially raised today. The biggest drawback to their use is the way they look. Frankly, they disgust most patients. Another potential problem is that leeches tend to wander off if left unattended. They have been known to disappear into rectums, uteri, and air passageways. In 1993, one wayward leech abandoned its duties of sucking the blood at the site of a breast reconstruction and crawled between the stitches holding the incision together and into the woman's breast.[3]

With these downsides in mind, researchers at the University of Wisconsin, Madison, developed a mechanical leech. It looks like a small bottle attached to a suction cup. It delivers an anticlotting agent to the damaged tissue and sucks out as much blood as needed. It has the added benefit of never getting full.

Is there such a thing as a 3-foot leech? (and other leech trivia)

- Most leeches are about 1 inch long, but some giants can grow to 3 feet.
- Medicinal leeches have three jaws that look like little saws studded with about 100 sharp teeth to cut into the skin.

- A leech may swell up to 10 times its normal size in one feeding.
- After a good blood meal, a leech can go for 9 months without another.

What condition causes your extremities to rot and fall off?

Gangrene is the death of body tissue from infection or lack of blood flow. It is most common in the extremities. There are two kinds of gangrene: dry and gas. Dry gangrene is caused by an interruption of blood flow not due to bacterial infection. Those affected by impaired peripheral blood flow, such as people with diabetes, are prone to dry gangrene. Symptoms include a coldness and achiness in the affected area and pallid flesh, followed by death of the tissue.

Gas gangrene results from a bacterial infection that produces gas within the affected tissues. It is usually caused by the *Clostridium perfringens* bacterium. The gas produced quickly expands and separates the tissues, allowing the bacteria to rapidly spread. The bacteria secrete strong toxins that cause sepsis and go on to poison the blood, inducing shock. Gas gangrene is deadly and is considered a medical emergency.

The best way to treat gangrene is to restore the blood flow to the damaged tissues. Failing that, debridement (removing the damaged tissue) with maggots is a good

option. (Maggots are discussed next.) Two less than
ideal alternatives are amputation and auto-amputation
(letting the tissue just fall off).

Are fly maggots really used to clean wounds?

If you ever broke open a trash bag containing your
kitchen garbage that had been left outside during the
hot summer months, you probably know what fly maggots are. These may be the most disgusting bugs on
Earth; but, yes, they are a valuable tool used by doctors
in the treatment of wounds. A maggot, as you should
know, is the larva of a fly, just as a caterpillar is the larva
of a moth. It has been known for centuries that maggots can heal wounds. Military surgeons noticed that
soldiers whose wounds became infested with maggots
healed better and had a lower mortality rate. William
Baer of Johns Hopkins University in Baltimore was the
first American surgeon to promote maggot débride-
ment therapy (MDT), its fancy name.

During World War I, Baer treated a soldier who had
been wounded and left on the battlefield for a few days.
The soldier had sustained a compound fracture to the
femur and massive flesh wounds to the abdomen and
scrotum. When the patient arrived at the hospital, he
had no fever, which was unheard of for the types of
wounds he had. When Baer removed the soldier's uniform he found thousands of maggots feeding on the

man's wounds. To the doctor's astonishment, there was no bare bone to be found, and the wounded areas were covered with healthy pink tissue. This is because some maggots eat only dead flesh and leave live flesh alone.

MDT was used routinely until the mid-1940s, when antibiotics and improved surgical techniques replaced the use of maggots. In the 1970s and 1980s, MDT was occasionally used when traditional modern surgical methods failed. In 1989, physicians at the Veterans Affairs Medical Center in Long Beach, California, and at the University of California at Irvine had the revelation that using maggots was good for wounds that didn't respond to other treatments.

Of the thousands of species of flies, some are better at MDT than others. One that has been used successfully for decades is the green blowfly (*Phaenicia sericata*). Blowflies lay their eggs and feed on dead or rotting flesh. They are usually the first insects attracted to a fresh carcass, sometimes arriving within minutes of death. They are attracted by the organic odors of death.

Thousands of clinics use these gross "worms" for cleaning, disinfecting, and promoting healing of many types of wounds, including bed sores, diabetic ulcers, and surgical wounds. The maggots are contained for 2 days in a special cage-like dressing, with the wound acting as the floor of the cage. There is a little window in the top of the dressing so the maggots can breathe and doctors can observe the proceedings within.

Countless limbs have been saved and cases of gangrene prevented thanks to green blowfly maggots. The bugs are also especially adept at treating bone infections. Because bones don't have a strong supply of blood, antibiotics have trouble getting there. Fortunately, maggots don't.

Where do doctors get blowfly maggots?

The only producer of green blowfly maggots is Monarch Labs, in Irvine, California. MDT larvae must be maintained germ-free and starving. Medical maggots are very perishable. They are produced daily from fresh fly eggs and must be shipped to the customer within 48 hours and used within 24 hours. Monarch Labs is capable of supplying up to 1 million maggots a week.

How was human skin used by bookbinders?

This would be considered an outrage today, but up until about 200 years ago some books were bound with human skin, especially medical books. In the days of yore, many doctors who wrote medical volumes specified that the binder use human skin. One notable example is a book by Englishman John Hunter (1728–1793), the father of British scientific surgery, who wrote a tome on, you guessed it, dermatology.

Where did one get skin for bookbinding? Most material came from executed murderers. In 1821, a John

Horwood was hung for murder, and his skeleton was displayed at the Bristol Royal Infirmary, in England. Also at the infirmary was a copy of a book detailing his crime, trial, execution, and dissection and it was bound, that's right, in Horwood's skin.

Many people willingly allowed their skin to be used for bindings. Some people who left their bodies to medicine signed off on the idea before their passing. It was not unheard of for someone to specify in a will that, after death, his or her skin be used to bind a special book to be presented to loved ones.

If you care to see some surviving copies of such works, the Cleveland Public Library, Harvard Law School, and Brown University all have excellent examples. One such tome is Andreas Vesalius's sixteenth-century anatomy book, *De Humani Corporis Fabrica, or On the Fabric of the Human Body,* bound in the fabric of the human body.

How can rubber bands be used to treat hemorrhoids?

Hemorrhoids, as you may or may not know, are inflammations and swellings in the veins of the rectum and anus. They are extremely common. Between 50 and 85 percent of the world's population will be affected at some time. Usually, they are not a big problem, but every year about 500,000 Americans seek medical attention for "piles," as they are also known.

Two common causes of hemorrhoids are straining

too hard while taking a dump or just sitting too much. Pregnant women are also very prone. Squatting while pooping may reduce the risk of piles. Studies have shown that in countries where people use squat toilets, hemorrhoids are very rare. One alternate method of defecating to avoid hemorrhoids is to go standing up with the legs slightly bent. This position uses the abdominal muscles to move the bowels, putting less strain on the anus (but makes reading the newspaper much more difficult).

There are two types of hemorrhoids. Internal hemorrhoids are not painful and most people don't even know they have them. To find internal hemorrhoids, a doctor will use an anoscope, which is basically a hollow tube with a light attached. You know where it goes.

External hemorrhoids are the ones that protrude outside of the anus. External hemorrhoids are easy to see and aren't exactly a pretty sight.

The treatments for piles are numerous. Severe hemorrhoids can be treated by any of a number of surgical methods, the most interesting being rubber band ligation. A rubber band is fastened around an internal hemorrhoid to cut off its blood supply. This causes the tissue to wither and die, after which it is carried away by a bowel movement. Cryosurgery can be used to freeze external hemorrhoids before removal. Products like Preparation H contain hydrocortisone, which reduces the swelling and itching.

Are some babies born with tails?

All human fetuses have something that resembles a tail, up until the eighth week of development. Fetuses also have gill slits that disappear well before birth. Some scientists think these are throwbacks to our early evolution from our more primitive animal ancestors. Be that as it may, it is the rare baby that is born with a tail.

The "tail," or caudal appendage as it's known, can be bony or fatty. A baby was born in India in 2001 with a 10-centimeter fatty tail. Named Balaji, he was worshipped by the locals as a reincarnated Hindu god and paid money to appear in their temples. In 2004, a Cambodian girl was born with an equally long tail.

Babies born with tails in the Western world have them snipped off at birth. No one is the wiser.

Can newborns lactate?

If you've ever had a baby, you probably know this one. Some babies are born with swollen breasts and a lump under the nipple about the size of a marble, or smaller. If squeezed, the lumps may exude something called "witches' milk." This is a sweet, whitish fluid that actually is milk. Shortly after birth, newborns are still under hormonal influence from their mothers. The hormones in the baby's blood can cause the glands in their breasts to lactate for up to a couple of weeks, even in baby boys.

Doctors advise against massaging or squeezing the breast lumps. This may introduce bacteria into the milk glands, causing an infection.

In the old days, midwives would collect witches' milk, believing that it possessed some magical properties. It was thought to cure infertility, among other sexual problems.

Why is your belly button so sensitive?

The abdominal wall is composed of several layers—muscle, fat, and skin. These three layers are all fused together at this one point. In essence, there is no subcutaneous fat under your navel. The skin is joined directly to your abdominal wall, with subcutaneous fat all around the navel. This is why your belly button is concave, if you have an "innie." "Outies" are caused by a protuberant mass of scar tissue between the abdominal wall and the navel, creating a convex belly button.

Many people report a tingly sensation when they touch their navels. In women it is more commonly reported as a pleasurable feeling, sometimes even stimulating their clitoris. Men more often experience unpleasant feelings, oftentimes in their penis. There is no hard proof, but it seems that nerves in the belly button correspond to genital stimulation centers in the brain.

How does belly button lint get in there?

Speaking of belly buttons, how is it that they seem to be lint magnets for some people? The navel, while cute to look at, serves no useful purpose. Happily, it requires very little maintenance, aside from the occasional lint cleaning. But how does that stuff get in there?

Not everybody gets belly button lint. One survey found that only 66 percent of us do.[4] And it seems to be a guy thing: 73 percent of men report having it, compared to only 27 percent of females. These numbers hint at the cause of belly button fluff—hair.

Most men are much hairier than their female counterparts. Research has shown that the hairier you are, especially in the lower abdominal region, the more lint you will accumulate. There's something known as a "snail trail." This is a line of hair that grows in one direction from the pubic area up to the navel. Snail trails are more prevalent in men. Women tend to have pubic hair that is shaped like an inverted pyramid, with a distinct cutoff at the top. Men, on the other hand, have pubic hair that gradually tapers off as it grows toward the belly button—the snail trail.

How does all this affect the amount of fluff in your navel? Snail trails act as conduits for lint and dead skin cells to travel up from your pants and underwear into the belly button. Too hairy a snail trail will reduce lint movement, as will too little hair. Some women have light snail trails, so they will gather some lint. The hair around the navel then prevents the lint from working its way back out. People who are overweight have deeper belly buttons and are likely to collect more fluff. Conversely, thin people have less of a lint problem.

While any color is possible, blue is the most common color of navel fluff. Just look at your dryer's lint screen. This is because blue is such a popular color for clothing (think blue jeans).

There's a guy in Australia who's been collecting his fluff since 1984. Graham Barke has 2½ big jars' worth at this writing and plans to keep going until he has enough to stuff a pillow.[5] (Just so long as his life has meaning.)

Can you have your breasts enlarged through your belly button?

Women who dread scar tissue formation from having breast-augmentation surgery have a new option. Plastic surgeons now can make a cut in the navel, snake an endoscope up under the skin over the rib cage to the breasts, where they can cut into the breasts and insert rolled up breast implants that can be filled with saltwater.

Are there any real "wolfmen"?

Any decent circus sideshow has a "wolfman," some guy covered from head to toe in hair. The medical term for having excess body hair is *congenital generalized hyper-trichosis,* also known as "werewolf syndrome." There is a clan of 24 people from Loreto, Zacatecas, Mexico, who are famed for their prodigious hairiness and *do* work in circuses. The gene that turns off hair growth on their face doesn't work.

The women in the family are covered in a light to medium coating of hair. The men have heavy hair growth on every square inch of their bodies, except their palms and soles. Their faces are totally covered in thick black hair, resembling the mythical werewolves. Two of the males—Larry and Danny Ramos Gomez—actually did work for some time in sleazy sideshows, but they are now employed by the Mexican National Circus as headlining acrobats known as the "Wolf Boys."

How many people have webbed feet?

Webbed toes are a more common birth condition than you may have thought (if you have ever thought about it, that is). They occur in roughly 1 in 2,000 to 2,500 live births. The medical term for the condition of having webbed toes or fingers is *syndactyly.* There are various degrees of webbedness, ranging from partial to complete, the most frequent being a fusion of, or webbing between, the second and third toes. In some cases, the bones of adjacent digits are fused together.

While a little weird, webbed toes are merely a cosmetic problem. They do not impair any normal activities.

If you are thinking about *The Man from Atlantis,* there is no evidence that webbed feet are any kind of advantage when it comes to swimming. Webbed fingers can be more problematic because they may impair finger movements.

For several weeks early in life, a human fetus has webbed digits. It's not until the sixteenth week of development that an enzyme is produced that dissolves away the webbing. In some fetuses, the tissue does not dissolve away completely, leaving webbed fingers or toes.

Surgery can be performed to "correct" this condition. Because there is no medical basis for such an operation, doctors may not want to do it until the child is old enough to decide for himself or herself about its merits.

Many famous people have webbed toes, including Ashton Kutcher, Dan Aykroyd, and Marge Simpson.

Webbed feet are common in many sporting dog breeds, such as the Labrador Retriever, Otterhound, Newfoundland, Field Spaniel, Irish Water Dog, and Nova Scotia Duck-Tolling Retriever—all water dogs.

How many people are born with extra fingers?

The rate of polydactylism (more than the normal number of fingers or toes) is greater than the rate of syndactyly, or webbed feet, which is approximately 1 in 1,000 live births. In the United States, the frequency of extra digits is higher in the Asian American and Amish populations. The most common type of extra digit is that of a small piece of soft tissue. This is easily treated in the nursery by tying a suture tightly around the base of the extra digit, causing it to fall off.

There may be bone inside the extra digit, and rarely a fully jointed finger or toe may be present. The extra digit is usually a fork in an existing digit. It is commonly found on the pinky side of the hand or foot, more rarely the thumb side or among the other digits. Surgery for the condition is common.

Why do old people have such big ears?

Have you ever been stuck behind a slow driver and wondered why he or she is plodding along at a snail's pace? Then you see the hat and the enormous ears sticking out, and it all becomes clear: An elderly gentleman is impeding your progress.

There seems to be something of a debate in the scientific community about why older people have large ears. Some say the rest of the body withers in old age, not the ears, so they just seem to be gargantuan. Others point out that the earlobe cartilage softens up later in life and that old people's ears aren't any bigger, just floppier and "stick-outier." Still other ear size scholars reckon our ears just keep on a growin' till we die, meaning they really are huge on old folks. Several recent research studies suggest that they do indeed get a little longer every year, not wider though.[6] The ear gains about 0.22 millimeters in length per year of life (and the driving gets a little slower).

When was brain surgery done with stone tools?

When you think of brain surgery, you think of high-tech science. However, the oldest known surgery is something called "trephination," an ancient surgery that involved the opening of the skull. In fact, trephined human skulls have been found that are over 10,000 years old. These operations were conducted for medical as well as for ritual reasons. Although skull trephination was performed in various areas around the world, it was in Bolivia and Peru the practice really flourished.

The procedure involved the removal of a piece of the skull to expose the dura mater (the tough fibrous membrane that envelopes the brain). When this was done properly, the dura mater remained intact and the "patient" had a good chance to survive without brain infection. Over two-thirds of ancient trephined skulls found show signs of healing, which indicates survival.

There were three basic methods that were employed: scraping, drilling, and cutting. Scraping and cutting involved using a flint or obsidian knife to scrape or cut repeatedly deeper circular or square-shaped grooves in the skull until the dura mater was reached. The etched-out piece of skull could then be pried off.

Drilling involved using a bow drill, in which a bow

made of springy wood had a leather cord wound around a drill (a wooden shaft with a sharp point) several times. The surgeon placed the tip of the drill on the head and spun it with the bow, much as native peoples do to start fires. After a series of holes were drilled in a circular pattern, the walls between the holes were then broken and a round piece of skull could be removed.

During the Middle Ages and the Renaissance in Europe, trephination was performed to treat skull fractures and seizures. Remarkably, it is still performed today in parts of Africa, South America, and Melanesia. Some pseudo-scientists still proclaim its virtues.

Who did the first human vivisections?

A Greek named Herophilus (335–280 BCE) is considered the father of anatomy. He was the first doctor to draw conclusions about the human body from direct observations—that is, vivisection. He made groundbreaking discoveries in the study of the nervous system, as well as many other parts of the body. Herophilus introduced many of the terms still used today to describe anatomical phenomena. Apparently, he was very thorough in his research. He reportedly vivisected over 600 live prisoners.

Two *more* notorious instances of human vivisection occurred during World War II. Both the Nazis, under Josef Mengele, and the Japanese military Unit 731, under

Fukujiro Ishiyama at Kyushu Imperial University Hospital, conducted human experiments, including vivisection of their respective concentration camp prisoners.

Who was the first guy to fill a cavity?

Does the sound of the dentist's drill send a chill up/down your spine? Just be glad you didn't have a guy named Rhazes filling your cavities. Rhazes, a tenth-century Persian physician, was, in fact, the first person to drill out the gunk from a cavity and fill in the hole. His drill was crude to say the least. It consisted of a metal spike that he spun back and forth between his thumb and forefinger. It must have been agonizingly slow. Once the horror of drilling out a hole was over, Rhazes filled it in with a glue-like paste of alum and mastic (a yellow tree resin). Rhazes's drilling technique lasted for 700 years, which explains why most people didn't get their cavities filled. By the late 1700s, dentists had devised a somewhat faster drill that could be hooked up to the spinning wheel found in homes of the time, but it must have still seemed excruciatingly slow.

Did George Washington wear donkey teeth dentures?

George Washington was the perhaps the greatest American ever. But he is most remembered for cutting down a cherry tree and wearing wooden dentures, neither of which he actually did. Washington, however, did have terrible dental problems. He started losing his teeth in his 20s. By the time he became president, he had only one of his own teeth left. George went through many sets of false teeth, but he never had wooden teeth. He finally had a good set of choppers made in 1798, from a denture plate of hippopotamus ivory to which human teeth, along with parts of donkey and horse teeth, were fitted. (Rumor has it that some of his replacement teeth came from his slaves.) His upper and lower dentures were connected with springs to help them open and close.

Such were his dental woes that when he sat for his official presidential portrait with the great artist Gilbert Stuart, his false teeth hurt so badly that he took them out. Stuart had poor George stuff cotton in his cheeks and lips to fill them out a little. If you grab a $1 bill, you'll notice just how puffy George's cheeks look.

What were the teeth of corpses used for?

Dental hygiene is a relatively recent development. For most of human history, people's teeth have been rotting and falling out of their heads. Around 700 BCE, the Etruscans were making beautiful artificial teeth. These dentures were made from hippopotamus, walrus, and elephant ivory. Human teeth were also used as replacements. Teeth were taken from corpses and poor people would pull their own for sale. Alas, these used human teeth did not last long, usually rotting and decaying in short order. The wealthy had replacement teeth fashioned from gold, silver, agate, or mother-of-pearl.

In medieval times, the art of denture making was lost, and folks just lived their lives with gaps in their smile. Even Queen Elizabeth I resorted to sticking bits of white cloth between her teeth when going out in public. When false teeth were fitted, they were hand carved and tied in place with silk threads. In 1774, porcelain dentures were developed. Plaster of Paris was used to make a mold of the person's mouth to which the dentures could be formed. Yet they didn't catch on right away.

During the 1800s, teeth were regularly plundered from the dead combatants on major battlefields. Most notably, thousands of teeth were collected after the Battle of Waterloo and shipped back to England to adorn the upper-class smile. While artificial teeth finally became popular in the 1840s, demand for human teeth was still big in the 1860s. Countless teeth from the American Civil War battlefields found their way into English mouths.

The invention of vulcanized rubber provided a soft, pliable base to hold the dentures, which could be shaped to fit the mouth. Today, dentures are made from a combination of porcelain, resin, metal, plastic, and ceramic.

Are some people blue?

In the early days of the nineteenth century, a French orphan named Martin Fugate, who was a carrier of an extremely rare recessive gene for a condition known as "hereditary methemoglobinemia," married a woman named Mary Smith who also carried the same rare gene. They settled down to live on the banks of Troublesome Creek, in eastern Kentucky. This incredibly rare match led to offspring who were quite bizarre. Four of the Fugate children were born with light blue skin, which they had for their entire lives.

It wasn't until a century later that scientists figured out what caused their bluish hue. Due to an enzyme deficiency, the Fugates' blood had a lowered oxygen-carrying capacity. Being somewhat isolated, they inbred over the years, resulting in many more blue Fugates. Six generations later, there were still blue Fugates to be found in the hills of eastern Kentucky.

Can coconut milk be used for blood plasma?

If you think this sounds nutty (sorry), read on. Coconuts are the most economically important nuts in the world. They are prized for their pulp, milk, oil, fiber, and wood. The word *coconut* derives from the Portuguese *coco,* meaning "goblin" or "monkey." The coconut's hard, dark brown hairy husk has three indentations on one end that somewhat resemble a monkey's face. In

Sanskrit, the coconut palm is known as *kalpa vriksha*, meaning "tree that gives all that is necessary for living," because nearly every part of the tree can be used for some practical purpose.

The milk contains coconut fat, which is chemically similar to butterfat and can be substituted for cow's milk for almost all cooking needs. The meat was used as a sweetener before sugar found widespread use. Dried coconut meat is pressed to extract coconut oil, which is used in a multitude of products, ranging from candies to cookies to cosmetics. Coconut palm fibers and wood have been used for millennia for everything from building materials to cooking fires. But perhaps the most amazing use for a coconut is that coconut water can be used as an emergency replacement for blood plasma. (This is good to know if you are ever on a desert island.)

If you have ever opened a fresh, young coconut, you have seen the watery, opaque coconut "water" inside. Contrary to popular belief, this is not coconut milk, which is made by boiling coconut meat in water. Coconut water is consumed as a fresh drink. It is more nutritious than whole milk, has less fat, is low in calories, and contains no cholesterol. Coconut water is also sterile; and, remarkably, it is a natural isotonic beverage, with the same electrolytic balance as that found in human blood. (It is marketed as a sports drink in some places.) What this means is that coconut water is a good natural source of blood plasma in a pinch.

Coconut water saved many lives in World War II. Both sides in the Pacific battles used coconut water transfusions, siphoned directly from the coconut into the wounded troops. This wonder beverage continues to save lives today in many third world countries, where coconut IVs are used.

Why do bruises turn yellow and green?

When you first get a simple bruise (which you can call a "contusion" if you want to make it to sound more serious), your skin typically first turns reddish. This is a result of trauma to muscle or other tissue just below the skin's surface. Ruptured capillaries bleed into surrounding tissue. Within hours, a purplish, or black and blue, color develops. The reason for the initial color change is hemoglobin. Fresh blood is bright red because of oxygen-carrying hemoglobin. Hemoglobin quickly loses oxygen when it seeps into tissues and begins to appear bluish. That much makes sense, but why does the black and blue turn green and yellow? Again, the answer is blood chemistry.

Within days or weeks, as a bruise continues to heal, the body breaks down the hemoglobin, using its iron to make new red blood cells. The remaining hemoglobin decomposes into a green pigment—biliverdin—that is further converted into a yellowish brown pigment called bilirubin. The result of these chemical reactions beneath your skin is that rather distasteful-looking multicolored blotch that gives many people the shivers. Eventually, the body reabsorbs all this nasty looking stuff and the skin returns to normal.

What condition can give you a bump the size of a bowling ball on your neck?

A goiter, or bronchocele, is a swelling of the throat or neck caused by iodine deficiency. Some of these babies can get quite large, approaching the size of a bowling ball. They used to be common before the days of iodized salt and iodine-supplemented foods. Today, goiter is found only in the poorest countries of central Africa, central Asia, and India, although it once was prevalent in the American Midwest, Great Lakes, and Intermountain regions. Some goiters are caused by an autoimmune problem that is more common in women.

How do they do a liposuction?

Liposuction is one of the most common plastic surgeries. But unless you've had it done or have watched it performed on the Learning Channel, you may not realize just how gross it is. In a nutshell, liposuction, as the name implies, is a procedure in which you have extra fat sucked out of your body with a special vacuum device. Liposuctions are generally done to flabby areas of the body—the abdomen, buttocks, thighs, and back of the arms. Women most often have their tummy and thighs vacuumed out; men have their beer guts and love handles reduced.

The first liposuctions were performed in the United States in the mid-1980s. General anesthesia was typically required. The original procedure was more dangerous than today's. It involved larger incisions and the insertion of longer hollow vacuum tubes (cannulas). One modern technique is called "tumescent liposuction." Smaller incisions and cannulas are employed under local anesthesia.

Tumescent means "swollen and firm," which is how the technique prepares the tissue for removal. A saline solution of lidocaine and epinephrine is injected into the fatty tissue. The lidocaine numbs the fat and causes it to swell up and become firm. The epinephrine helps reduce bleeding. Large amounts of this fluid are used to create space between the muscle and fatty tissue, making more room for the suction tube. Manual effort is required to pulverize the fat for suction.

Alternately, ultrasound can be used to implode and liquefy the fat, turning it into a yellowish mush before it is sucked out. This method targets fat cells specifically, causing less blood and tissue loss.

Fat deposits adhere to the underside of the skin and can be removed if they can be dislodged. After numbing the area, small incisions are made and cannulas are slipped in the cuts and vigorously scraped around under the skin to loosen the fat. It's quite disgusting to watch. The tubes then suck the fat away. Large areas of fat can be numbed and sucked out using this technique. The lidocaine remains in the tissue for up to 36 hours, reducing postsurgery pain.

Can human fat be recycled?

Thousands of liposuction patients a year literally have the fat sucked out of their bodies. Where does all this disgusting goo go? Most of it is chucked out, but one enterprising Miami businessperson sees a pot of gold in goop. Lauri Vernoy has a deal with Jackson Memorial Hospital in Miami to recycle 3,000 gallons of human fat a week from the clinic's liposuction procedures. Vernoy says that is enough to produce 2,600 gallons of biodiesel. If there's one thing that is not in short supply, it's cellulite. Watch out ExxonMobil!

How do people shrink heads?

There aren't many things more creepy than a shrunken head. They aren't easy to make. Only an expert can do it. Most of these experts live in the jungles of Brazil, Peru, and Ecuador. They are the Jivaro people, best known for what they do to their enemies' heads. Since about 200 BCE, they have been raiding other tribes to obtain *tsantsas,* or shrunken head trophies. Typically, a Jivaro warrior will target just one hut and take the head of any man, woman, or child caught unaware. A male warrior's head is preferred because this trophy will give one more prestige and fill the taker with the victim's power. (Makes sense.)

So how does one shrink a head? Obviously, the head should first be removed from the body. The skin is cut back around the top parts of the chest and back and the head is cut off near the collarbone. A vine is then passed through the head to make carrying easier while beating a hasty retreat. On the trip home, which may take several days (one can't be loping off heads in the village next door), short stops are made to start preparing the head for downsizing.

The skin is slit at the back of the skull and carefully peeled off. The skull is then tossed into a river as a gift to the anaconda. After being boiled in water for about 30 minutes, the skin, which is now about half its original size, is put on a stick to dry. After drying, the skin is turned inside out and any remaining flesh is scraped off. It is turned right side out again and the mouth and the slit in the back are sewn shut. Sewing the eyes shut is optional—a matter of personal choice.

Hot rocks are repeatedly put inside the skin to further shrink it, followed by several treatments with hot sand. Placing the skin over a smoldering fire overnight will impart that ghoulish blackened appearance that is so desirable. Finally, the head is ready for shaping, and a hot knife is used to finish drying the lips. You now have an expertly fashioned shrunken head.

By this time, the warrior should be close to home and ready to enter his village with his trophy shrunken heads tied around his neck. This is when the *tsantsa* ritual party begins. What mom wouldn't be proud?

(Kids, please don't try this at home. The Jivaros *are* professionals.)

On a serious note, the governments in these countries had to crack down on the Jivaro because they started selling shrunken heads for profit to collectors from the outside world. This meant they had to kill more people than just those needed for traditional rituals. The sale of shrunken heads is currently banned worldwide. They are now made as curios for tourists from animal hides carved to resemble the real thing. How can you tell if you are buying an authentic shrunken head or a cheap knockoff? Check for nostril hair. Fakes don't have it. Caveat emptor.

Which culture used to bind the heads of babies between wooden boards?

The Chinese practice of binding young girls' feet to satisfy the male small foot fetish is well known. Fewer people are aware that the pre-Columbian Olmec civilization of south-central Mexico used to bind a royal baby's head between boards when he or she was 2 weeks old. An infant's skull bones are not yet fused and thus can be pressed into a tall shape if bound for their first 2 years of life. This made the head grotesquely elongated like that of the Coneheads of *Saturday Night Live* fame. There's no accounting for taste.

When were mummies used as medicine?

During the Middle Ages, some folks believed that mummies possessed properties of medicinal value. By the twelfth century, mummy powder was used to cure wounds and bruises. For 500 years, European "doctors" prescribed mummy powder. It wasn't just Egyptian mummies that were in demand. In 1402, after Spain invaded the Canary Islands, thousands of mummies were discovered there because the Guanche people of the islands once practiced mummy making.

When were varicose veins popular?

Although ladies today spend thousands of dollars to get rid of unsightly blue varicose veins, the Egyptians went to great lengths to enhance them. The wardrobe preference of the time consisted of translucent fabric draped over the body in various ways. The breasts may or may not have been exposed. Those that were covered were not well hidden. Either way, a lot of skin showed.

One feature that made a gal particularly proud of her bosom was the presence of dark blue veins. These were also quite desirable on the legs, which were often exposed. To enhance this sign of beauty, women would deepen the bluish color of their veins with dye.

When was female baldness in vogue?

Today, women treasure thick, luxuriant hair. This was not always the case. In Egypt, around 1500 BCE, a completely bald head was all the rage for women. Obtaining a cue-ball noggin was no easy matter back then. Sharp razors did not exist. The poor gal had to have her hairs plucked out of her scalp one by one with tweezers. The chrome dome would then be buffed to a high shine. (And you think plucking a few eyebrow hairs is painful.)

What antidepressant drug can give you an orgasm when you yawn?

This is another one of those questions that sounds like it's got to be made up. But the following cases come from the respected *Canadian Journal of Psychiatry*, not *Playboy* "Forum."[7]

Some women taking the antidepressant clomipramine (Anafranil) experienced spontaneous orgasms every time they yawned. Even deliberate yawning produced an orgasm. The drug, which is supposed to elevate mood and boost physical activity, seems to go above and beyond that description for about 5 percent of the people taking it. Many women found the side effects quite pleasurable and wanted to stay on the drug after they no longer needed it for their psychological problems. (Can you blame them?)

Some men have reported the same experience, which can be somewhat embarrassing, as you may well imagine. Not only do they get a full-blown erection, but they ejaculate with no stimulation or sexual thoughts beforehand. Male patients taking clomipramine have resorted to wearing condoms throughout the day to keep from ejaculating in their shorts—a definite social faux pas.

Can anybody suck up water through their anus?

There once was a guy who became a professional at this somewhat unique talent. He was known as a "fartist," or "flautist." His stage name was Le Pétomane, from the French péter, "to fart," and –mane, "maniac."

His real name was Joseph Pujol (1857–1945). He had the unique ability to draw water up into his colon at will. He was able to then expel the water like a fountain through his anus to a distance of several yards. His classmates and army buddies were much impressed, so Pujol took his act to the stage in 1887. By 1892, he was performing at the Moulin Rogue in Paris. Some of his greater accomplishments were being able to blow out a candle several yards away, smoking a cigarette, and playing an ocarina (flute) through a rubber tube attached to his anus.

In 2006, a musical based on his life, *The Fartiste,* played in New York. There is a present-day imitator named Mr. Methane.

Was there ever a tumor removed that was bigger than the patient? (and other disgusting medical records)

- The largest gallstone ever removed was from an 80-year-old London man in 1952. This poor chap had a 131-pound, 8-ounce behemoth excised from his body.

- The largest tumor ever removed intact was a 303-pound monster (that's twice the size of many people!) taken from the right ovary of a 34-year-old woman in 1991. It took 6 hours on the operating table at the Stanford Medical Center to wrestle out the 3-foot, 3-inch mass. After the operation, the woman weighed *only* 210 pounds. She left the operating room on one stretcher; the tumor left on another.

- The biggest brain tumor ever removed came from a 4-year-old Indore, Indiana, girl and weighed 1 pound, 6 ounces.

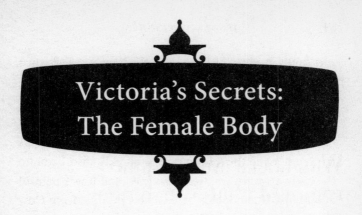

Victoria's Secrets: The Female Body

Artists have glorified the female body for millennia. In modern times, there is little about females that has not been written about extensively in the plethora of women's magazines. The following, however, is a collection of grotesque female facts that have escaped widespread coverage in the traditional pop culture media.

Why did women once have goat's milk and paraffin wax injected into their boobs?

American women weren't the first to try to enlarge the size of their boobs artificially. That would be the Japanese.

During the post–World War II occupation of Japan by American GIs, there was a flourishing prostitution trade. The working girls quickly discovered that Joe was more attracted to the girls with the bigger breasts, just like the girls back home. Unfortunately, most Japanese women had a more diminutive bosom. What to do?

They first tried having saline solution or goat's milk injected into their boobs. Any swelling of the breasts was temporary, and the solutions were quickly absorbed into the body. Paraffin wax was also tried, but it was painful and lumpy. Then doctors tried a new product from Dow Corning—silicone gel. It was used by the military and was easy to get on the black market. It was an instant hit.

Silicone was inert; was not absorbed into the body; had a soft, natural feel; and greatly increased the size of the bosom. It wasn't long before the wonders of this magical new breast-enhancing substance reached American plastic surgeons—and the rest, as they say, is history.

What leading American doctor once recommended suckling puppies?

This question is from the truth-is-stranger-than-fiction files. Born in Pottsgrove, Pennsylvania, in 1768, William DeWees was a famous obstetrician. A graduate of the University of Pennsylvania, DeWees devoted himself exclusively to the field of obstetrics, which was quite unusual back then. He had to overcome the objections of the medical community to physicians who practiced midwifery, but in doing so he made obstetrics a respected branch of medicine.

DeWees also wrote the first American pediatric guide, which was sorely needed. However, he may have offended the sensibilities of some of its readers when he recommended that a pregnant woman suckle puppies during her seventh month to help toughen the nipples! Apparently, the good doctor never tried this advice himself or it might have been omitted from his work.

What women *have* suckled puppies?

Although the advice of DeWees may have been ignored, there are some women who do suckle puppies. Wildlife expert Jack Hanna recently told CNN's Larry King that 4,000 to 5,000 years ago, Australian Aborigines took dingo puppies from their dens and had nursing women suckle them as their own.[1] This bonded the dingoes with the Aboriginal mother and made them easier to domesticate. As adults, after the dingoes hunted and killed a kangaroo, the dogs would go back to their "mother's" house (hut) to share the meat.

It is shocking that some modern-day women breast-feed puppies. In June 2006, new mother Kine Skiaker was saddened by the death of her Canarian Warren Hound after it gave birth to 10 puppies. The plucky Norwegian, against her vet's advice, took the pups to her own lactating breasts. She nursed the pups for a couple of days, along with her 3-month-old son, Emil, until foster homes were found for all 10. (Don't you just love happy endings?)

In 2004, a New Zealand woman, Kura "Kat" Turmanako, breast-fed her Staffordshire bull terrier pup for several weeks, after her 2½-month-old baby went on the bottle. She said her hope was that the dog would protect the baby as they grew up. Animal rights groups worried that doing so might cause the dog long-term behavioral problems. (With an owner like this, that's a given.)

How many women have extra nipples?

Nipples. We all have them, but usually in pairs. Some gals (about 2 percent) have an added "bonus," however—an extra nipple. These are known as "supernumerary" nipples. Mostly they are small and kinda resemble a freckle or a mole. They occur along the "milk lines," which run down from under the armpits, through the regular nipples, and end near the groin. In about 5 percent of reported cases, the extra nipple is found outside the milk line, on the back, shoulder, limbs, vulva, or even the face.

There are eight degrees of development recognized for supernumerary nipples—from a simple patch of hair, all the way to a fully developed extra breast in miniature. The condition of having an extra nipple is known as "polythelia"; "polymastia" denotes the rarer condition of having an extra breast. In a few cases, supernumerary nipples can even lactate during pregnancy. What's more, in extremely rare cases, some women have had up to 10 functional breasts! Many women wear their extra nipples with pride, but others have them removed.

Rumor has it that Henry VIII's second wife, Ann Boleyn, had a third breast and six fingers on each hand. Alas, even these "enhancements" couldn't save her from the Tower of London. They were used against her as evidence of witchcraft at her trial in 1536.

More seldom, men can also have extra nipples. Witness singer/actor Mark Wahlberg, who has one below his left normal one. In a rare condition in men, called "gynecomastia," the poor guy grows several enlarged breasts.

Do women have sperm ducts?

No, not real ones anyway. It takes 6 or 7 weeks after fertilization for the human embryo to sexually differentiate. At this time, the hormones estrogen or testosterone kick in and send the fetus on its way to maleness or femaleness. Women have an epoophoron, a cluster of useless cells near the ovaries that would have become the male vas deferens, or sperm ducts, had not estrogen intervened.

What saint had her breasts cut off?

There is not too much information about this saint. Her name was Agatha and she lived in Italy during the first half of the third century. Legend has it that she was a pretty, young Christian girl, who led a chaste life, devoted to God. The local magistrate—Quinctianus—was a feared persecutor of Christians. He tried to coerce Agatha into sex under the threat of persecution. When she refused, he had her beaten and forced her to work in a brothel. After she refused to service any customers, Quinctianus had her breasts cut off and left her to bleed to death. She experienced a vision of St. Peter coming to her and bandaging her wounds. When Quinctianus discovered that Agatha had survived, he had her stretched on the rack and then rolled in hot embers. As she was being tortured, an earthquake occurred which scared off her tormenters. After thanking God for ending her pain, Agatha died.

Today, locals believe that carrying her death veil in a procession will keep Mt. Etna from erupting. She is the saint for preventing volcanic eruptions. Agatha is also the patron saint of wet nurses, rape victims, and breast diseases. Her representation is breasts on a dish, and her feast day is February 5, if you wish to observe.

Where in the world do women have abnormally large buttocks?

There is a medical condition known as "steatopygia," wherein the buttocks and thighs produce copious amounts of excessive fat. This condition is common among the Hottentot people of southern Africa, the Bushmen, and the pygmies of central Africa, especially the women. Fat development begins in young girls soon after birth and is completed after puberty.

Some members of the Hottentot tribe can have buttocks in which each half spans some 2 to 3 feet. Steatopygia is even nicknamed after them—"Hottentot apron." Happily, this culture considers a huge butt as a great sign of beauty.

Steatopygia is often associated with another condition known as elongated labia, wherein the labia minor (inner lips of the vulva) can hang down as much as 4 inches from the vulva.

Anthropologists believe that such a condition was fairly common among our ancient ancestors. Prehistoric ivory figures have been found in French caves that seem to show abnormally large thighs and elongated labia. Evolutionarily speaking, excessive amounts of stored fat helped these African women continue to reproduce during seasonal droughts and other times of food scarcity. The protruding backside also allows a child to rest on the women's back while she does work. Most convenient.

What women intentionally lengthen their labia?

Two different African tribes—the Venda of southern Africa and the Benin of western Africa—value elongated labia (vaginal lips). Because this state does not occur naturally, what's a girl to do? At a young age, the girls begin tugging on their labia. If they get tired, they have a friend do some tugging for them. In time, a mature Venda or Benin woman's lips may hang down some 7 inches! What does a busy lady do with dangling labia while she's trying to get all her chores done? Simple. She just folds them up into the vagina. Problem solved!

There are also some women in the Eastern Caroline Islands—the Ponapeans—who favor elongated labia and clitorises. Their method of achieving this condition is somewhat more painful. They rub stinging ants on their privates!

Why did some women used to put garlic in their vaginas?

The fair maidens of the 1500s placed cloves of garlic in their vaginas to test for fertility. They mistakenly believed that after 12 hours' time, if the woman's breath smelled of garlic, she was fertile.

Why did women used to put dung in their vaginas?

Since the dawn of humankind, women have sought to control pregnancy. Today, we would be repulsed by the thought of a woman putting dung in her vagina, but such were the lengths to which a woman would go in ancient times to prevent an unwanted pregnancy. Egyptian women concocted a paste of crocodile dung and inserted it into their vaginas. They thought that this would block the passage of sperm. It also probably discouraged all but the most ardent admirers from penetration.

Another interesting Egyptian contraceptive concoction involved mixing sodium carbonate (a salt) with honey or gum. Cloths soaked in honey with acacia tips were likewise used. In India, honey was also used to prevent pregnancies. It was combined with things like clarified butter, oils, and rock salt. The Greeks used cedar and olive oils, mixed with frankincense and lead, to good effect. Salts and lactic acid, as found in acacia, stop sperm dead in their tracks. Lactic acid is still used in spermicides. Elephant dung, which is very high in lactic acid, was used successfully by the Muslims. These early contraceptives may actually have worked. The ancients didn't understand the science, but they recognized when something was effective. Gooey stuff, like honey, does indeed slow down sperm motility.

Other cultures took less successful, albeit very creative approaches. The Jews, who believe, according to the Torah, that man is to be fruitful and multiply, left birth control up to the women. They relied on a combination of sponges, herbal teas, and jumping up and down after intercourse. The Romans would put pepper in their vaginas and sneeze a lot. During the Middle Ages, women depended more on superstition. One humorous contraceptive practice was to spit three times into the mouth of a frog after doing it.

Why did Egyptian women pee on wheat seeds?

No, pee is not a good fertilizer. Ancient women, like ladies today, needed a reliable way to determine if they were with child. Around 4,000 years ago, Egyptian doctors had women place wheat and barley seeds in a cloth and pee on it daily. If both kinds of seeds germinated, the gal was pregnant. If the highly prized wheat seeds sprouted first, she was to be blessed with a son. If the lowly barley seeds germinated first, she was to have a less-desirable daughter.

Although their science made no sense at all, it is curious that they made the connection between changes in the urine and being pregnant. Today's at-home early pregnancy tests are more reliable, but even they can't predict the sex of the baby.

How are frogs used to test for pregnancy?

Simple. Inject some urine into the dorsal lymph sac of a South African clawed frog and wait 8 to 12 hours. A dose of a pregnant woman's pee will cause the female frog to lay eggs. Likewise, a male frog will produce sperm in response to the injection.

The test works because a pregnant woman's urine contains a hormone called human chorionic gonadotropin (hCG). Modern at-home pregnancy test kits use antibodies to detect hCG. Until the 1960s, the only reliable way to test for pregnancy was to inject pee into an animal and wait for a reaction.

A test using rabbits was developed in 1927 and became known as the "rabbit test." A woman's pee was injected into live rabbits. After one to several days, the rabbits were dissected and their ovaries examined for changes. A common misconception is that the rabbit would die only if the woman was pregnant, hence the euphemism "the rabbit died," meaning the test was positive. Unfortunately, all the rabbits died, as they had to be cut open to be examined. They could have been stitched back up and nursed back to health, but this would not have been cost-effective. Oh well.

Another interesting pregnancy test employing animals was the "Bitterling test." This test was used during the 1800s in eastern Europe. It involved putting a carp-like fish into a quart of water with 2 teaspoons of a woman's pee. If the hormones in her urine made the oviducts of the fish descend, the woman was pregnant.

Why would a woman in the Middle Ages put a live fish in her vagina?

The things some women will do to arouse a man! Ladies during the Dark Ages were known to put a live fish in their vagina and leave it there until it died. Then they would cook it and serve it up to make their man amorous.

Failing this, a medieval woman might also try the sure-fire method of making an imprint of her vulva on a loaf of bread before baking. (Now you know why they were called the Dark Ages.)

Can a woman have her vagina tightened?

In a procedure called "female genitalia enhancement," fat is removed from the thighs, emulsified, and injected into the outer labia. They are then squeezed to reposition the fat up into the vaginal walls. A successful operation will result in a woman feeling much tighter to her partner and him feeling much bigger to her. A win-win situation if there ever was one.

What is a queef?

A *queef* is a female "fart" that, shall we say, comes out an orifice a man does not possess. Air sometimes gets trapped up there. Women who make love on all fours, among other ways, often introduce air into their vaginas in the process. When they move certain ways, it comes out with a farting kind of noise. Some women are able to control their vaginal muscles enough to queef at will.

What's the grossest thing ever found in a woman's privates?

This is a judgment call of course, but a report in the *American Journal of Forensic Medicine and Pathology*, in 1990, seems to win the prize.[2] An unnamed 29-year-old woman went to see her doctor regarding missed periods and wanting to terminate a pregnancy. The physician found and removed a 7-centimeter-long by 3-centimeter-in-diameter "cylindrical mass of pale-gray tissue" from her vagina. Upon questioning her, the doctor determined that it was an old deer tongue that she had used to masturbate with some time earlier and somehow forgotten! This stuff is too gross to make up.

Why did women douche with Lysol during the Depression?

Warning: Do Not Try This at Home!!! The word *douche* comes from the French, meaning to "wash or soak." It is estimated that 20 to 40 percent of American women aged 15 to 44 years douche regularly. About half of these women douche every week. Reasons for douching include general vaginal maintenance, cleaning away blood after monthly periods, getting rid of odors, killing sexually transmitted diseases, and preventing pregnancy. Douching is good for none of these, and most doctors recommend against it. No such advice was available 80 years ago.

The vagina, like a modern-day oven, is self-cleaning. When you douche, you kill the good vaginal bacteria that keep your vagina healthy. This allows bad bacteria to grow in their absence, causing infections.

During the 1920s, American women had very little reliable information on birth control. Some were desperate enough to try anything, including disinfectants! Magazine ads of the time promoted Lysol as a female douche, in addition to being a household cleaner. Women used the stuff to disinfect the toilet, then as a post-intercourse douche to kill sperm (now that's a wonder product). Some used it to excess (if a little is good, a lot must be better) and ended up burning their cervix and vagina. Coca-Cola has also been used as a contraceptive douche in different parts of the world.

What people kept their umbilical cords in an amulet?

The Cheyenne and Sioux tribes put their baby's umbilical cords in beaded holders, which were kept as amulets to guarantee a long life. Western Sioux or Lakota mothers-to-be made two pouches, one shaped like a lizard and one shaped like a turtle. When her baby was born, she placed its umbilical cord inside one of these—the lizard if it was a boy and the turtle if it was a girl. A tribal priest would pray that the Creator give to a boy the qualities of the lizard (speed and the ability to change) and to girls the qualities of the turtle (long life and strength).

The Lakota kept these dried bits of tissue that once connected them to their mother all their life and then were buried with them.

Do some women create artwork with their placentas?

In some parts of the world, the umbilical cord and placenta are not cut, but are left on until they dry up and fall off. This is called a Lotus birth. Some cultures bury the placenta in the ground to give it back to the earth. A tree or flower is planted on the spot a year later to be sustained by the placental nutrients.

Another bizarre practice is called placenta art. The new mom, or a family member, lays the placenta out on a piece of paper and the blood and amniotic fluid stain it, creating a "placenta print" that can be framed and hung on the wall.

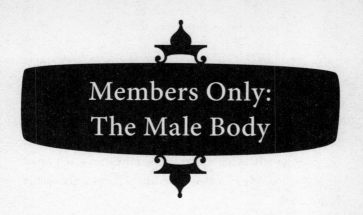

Members Only: The Male Body

The penis is a unique thing. No two are exactly the same. Whether or not a penis is an object of beauty is certainly a matter of personal taste. There are numerous conditions of the male member that are pretty weird and wild. Some of them you may be aware of, most of them you probably aren't. Here's a look at some of the grosser aspects of "man's best friend."

Do some penises have the hole on the lower side of the shaft?

One rather bizarre penile condition is hypospadias. It is a congenital disorder that can occur in 1 out of 400 to 500 infant penises. Unlike the normal penile configuration, in which the hole (urethral opening for you med students) is at the end, in hypospadias, the hole is on the lower side of the shaft. This condition can make urinating standing up rather tricky.

Surgery can be performed on the boy before he reaches school age. In it, a tube is created that extends to a new urethral opening at the tip of the penis. The old hole is left as is, since the urethra now bypasses it. The lad now has a two-holed penis, but only one is functional.

Can the foreskin get stuck behind the head of the penis?

Talk about painful. Phimosis is a tightening of the penis foreskin that prevents retraction over the glans (head) in uncircumcised males. It is a thin contour of skin tissue located near the front of the inner foreskin that narrows the opening of the foreskin. A phimotic ring can make retraction of the foreskin over and behind the glans difficult, painful, or impossible. The foreskin may even get stuck behind the glans. Circumcision is the easy solution to this problem.

Some historians believe that phimosis prevented Louis XVI of France from impregnating his wife—Marie Antoinette—for the first 7 years of their marriage. Another famous, or should we say infamous, person from history had phimosis—Charles Guiteau—the guy who assassinated President James Garfield in 1881. The coroner rather simplistically suggested that his murderous behavior was caused by "phimosis-induced insanity."

Some women suffer from a female version of this

condition, known as "vaginal phimosis." In it, the hood of skin surrounding the clitoris is too tight or there is no opening in the skin for the glans of the clitoris to protrude. This condition can result in a lack of sexual stimulation and sexual dysfunction.

What disorder can cause the penis to bend sideways when erect?

Peyronie's disease is a rare connective tissue disorder in men over 40, involving the formation of painful hard scar tissue, known as plaque, on one side of the penis. This hardened tissue causes the penis to bend distinctly to one side when erect. Sometimes the bend may be at an angle of 45 degrees, resulting in serious pain during erection and making normal intercourse impossible. It is curious that many men with Peyronie's disease report concurrent connective tissue problems in the hands or feet. In serious cases, surgery can correct the curvature, but at some cost. It usually shortens your member a little.

Can a man really get an erection that lasts more than 4 hours?

Priapism is a spontaneous, long-lasting erection over which the man has no control. Sound like a good thing?

No. It is very painful and may require surgically drain-
ing the blood away from the engorged penis through
tiny slits. A rare condition, priapism can be a somewhat
embarrassing side effect of male virility drugs. (If you've
noticed, their happy little commercials end by warning
you to see your doctor if you get an erection that lasts for
more than 4 hours.)

The word *priapism* comes from Greek mythology.
Aphrodite, the goddess of sex and love, had a son named
Priapus, the Greek god of fertility. He was blessed (or
cursed) with a perpetual erection.

Normally, a man gets an erection when the brain tells
the arteries that feed the corpus cavernosum, spongy
tissues that fill with blood during an erection, to dilate.
The spongy tissue that encapsulates the urethra and
the head of the penis also fill with blood and harden.
This constricts the veins leaving the penis, causing an
erection.

There are two types of priapism: nonischemic and
ischemic. Nonischemic priapism may result from an
injury to an artery that leads to the corpus cavernosum and may cause blood to spill into the erectile tissues. Because the rate of inflow may exceed the outflow
through the veins, a semirigid erection may result
which can last hours. An ice pack is generally sufficient
to resolve this problem.

Ischemic priapism results when blood flows into the
penis but doesn't flow back out. This loss of circulation
deprives the corpus cavernosum of oxygen and produces a painful, ultra-erection. Left untreated for more

than 12 hours, the erectile tissues can become damaged. In severe cases, gangrene can set in and amputation may be required. (No wonder the drug ads tell you to get to the doctor's office after 4 hours!) A urologist will need to make tiny cuts at the base of the penis to release the blood. He or she may also inject a saline solution to flush the blood out. If this does not work, drugs that constrict the arteries can be injected to stop the flow of blood into the penis. In rare cases, more drastic surgery is required.

The female counterpart to priapism is "clitorism," a long-lasting, painful erection of the clitoris.

Why does it hurt so much when a guy gets kicked in the groin?

The testicles are supersensitive because they are packed with nerve endings. The testes form in the abdomen, and the blood vessels and nerves remain attached there even after they descend. So a shot in the groin sends pain all the way into the pit of the stomach. Testicular trauma (the fancy name for getting hit in the balls) may cause a fella to throw up or even pass out.

One reason testicles swing freely and are such slippery little guys is to help them slide out of the way when hit by something hard.

Can you break an erection?

This must rank pretty high on the pain scale! Although an extremely rare occurrence, it is possible to break an erect penis. How, you may ask, does one break a boner? The most frequent causes are reported to be overenthusiastic masturbation and thrusting too hard during intercourse and accidentally smashing it into a woman's pubic bone. Other more bizarre ways are forcing it into a pair of tight jeans, rolling over on it the wrong way, and bumping it into a bedpost.

What are the symptoms of a broken erection? Well, obviously extreme pain comes first, followed by rapid swelling of the member to three to four times its normal circumference. Seeing a physician may be required to drain excess blood and repair damaged tissue.

Can a man have more than one penis?

Just as a woman, in rare cases, can have more then two breasts, a man can have more than one penis. Do you think this would be a blessing or a curse? Well, it's a curse. These poor guys are sterile. Only a few dozen cases of "diphallasparatus," as it's known, have ever been reported. Those afflicted can have the two penises one on top of the other or side by side. They will both be the same size and pee can come out of either one or both. (That's some weird and wild stuff.)

Why does a cold shower cause a man's genitals to shrivel up?

Perhaps nothing is more embarrassing for a man than to be caught unexpectedly after taking a cold shower. So what happens? Well, each testicle is suspended on a muscle called a cremaster that regulates the way it hangs. When the cremasters are relaxed, a man's balls hang low. When they contract, the cremasters will pull the testicles up, sometimes all the way into the inguinal area of the lower abdomen. This occurs when a man ejaculates. Cold, fear, fatigue, and excitement can also produce the phenomenon of the disappearing testicles. (Male readers should check their nuts the next time their team scores a touchdown in the big game.)

That explains the balls. Why does the penis shrink in cold water? Simple. The vessels that supply and inflate it with blood also contract when cold. It's kind of like how a balloon deflates on a cold day.

When did European men openly display their genitals?

One definite fashion no-no today is the display of the male member. Such was not the case in thirteenth-century Europe. Noblemen of the time were proud as peacocks, and happy to show off what they had. The fashion of the day called for the well-dressed gentleman to expose his genitals through an opening in the crotch of his tights. (Yes, guys wore tights back then.) Their tunics were waist length and didn't obstruct the view of the male splendor. Those gents not so well-endowed could wrap their package in a *braquette,* which was a flesh-colored, padded penis made of leather.

The fourteenth through sixteenth centuries were more modest times. Men then preferred to wear a codpiece, which was a protective penis sheath. (*Cod* is an Old English word meaning "scrotum.") The codpiece evolved from the metal crotch cover knights wore on their armor. In fashion, it was stuffed and ornately decorated, and worn with tight breeches. Tights in those days had a fly, but no zipper. Stuffing cloths in there also served the purpose of keeping Mr. Johnson from popping out. Because tights had no pockets, gents would keep their money, car keys, and credit cards in their codpiece. (Well, they would have if they'd had them.)

In the heyday of the codpiece, this fashion statement was taken to the extreme. Codpieces that protruded 5 inches were not uncommon. Finally, the Church had enough of this and condemned them as "fashions of the Devil." We can be thankful that they went the way of the dodo. Today's double-stitched trouser fly is a remnant of the old codpiece.

Can you have your penis lengthened?

Anything is possible through the wonders of modern science. Do you have an extra six grand lying around? That's about what you'll need. The penis-lengthening process is called "phalloplasty." Approximately one-third to one-half of the penis is inside the body and is attached to the underside of the pubic bone. The lengthening procedure involves releasing the suspensory ligaments that attach the penis to the pubic bone. This allows the surgeon access to the section of the penis hidden behind the skin wall. He or she then is able to extend the length of the penis in proportion to the internal portion, allowing the penis to protrude on a straighter path, farther outward, to provide more functional length. Specially designed penile weights are recommended by some doctors to maximize lengthening during the healing process. (Ouch!)

Depending on their anatomy, men can gain an extra 1½ to 2 inches in length. Overweight men can also have some fat removed from the pubic area. This will add to the "perceived" length increase of the penis.

Men can have girth increased, too, for another three grand. To boost the circumference by up to 50 percent, the surgeon can suck some fat cells from elsewhere on the body, inject them under the skin of the penis, and mold it into the proper shape.

Where is the world's only penis museum?

Yes, there actually is a museum devoted totally to penises; it's in Iceland. The Icelandic Phallological Museum in Iceland's capital—Reykjavik—houses 245 specimens in formaldehyde, dried, or displayed like hunting trophies. The collection represents almost all of Iceland's land and sea mammals, as well as some examples from other countries.

Some of the more bizarre displays include tanned bull penises that were once used as whips, a 3-foot whale penis, and smoked horse penises said to have been a favorite Icelandic snack in the 1930s. About 3,500 curiosity seekers wander into the museum each year at $4 a pop. The museum is hoping to acquire its first human penises soon. Some kindly gentlemen have recently willed their members to the place when they die.

The Russian Museum of Erotica opened in St. Petersburg, in 2004. Its claim to fame is the penis of the "Mad monk," Grigory Rasputin, whose unit measures some 30 centimeters (11.8 inches). The opening of the museum ended decades of Russian penis envy. The museum director is Igor Knyazkin, chief of the prostate research center at the Russian Academy of Sciences. He was quoted in the Russian daily *Nezavisimaya Gazeta* as saying before the grand opening, "Having this exhibit, now we can stop envying America, where Napoleon Bonaparte's penis is now kept. Napoleon's penis is but a small 'pod,' it can not stand in comparison to our organ of 30 centimeters."[1] (Bitter memories of the Napoleonic Wars apparently die hard.)

How many calories are there in semen?

Practitioners of fellatio out there may be happy to learn that semen is very low-cal. Only about 3 percent of semen is composed of sperm. The rest is seminal fluid, which contains 30 some odd chemicals, including blood group antigens, ascorbic acid, calcium, chlorine, cholesterol, citric acid, creatine, DNA, fructose, glutathione, hyaluronidase, inositol, lactic acid, nitrogen, phosphorus, potassium, pyruvic acid, sodium, sorbitol, spermidine, urea, uric acid, vitamin B_{12}, and zinc. Sounds like a lot of good stuff; but, alas, the nutrient value of semen is around zip. It does, however, nourish the sperm long enough to help them make their arduous journey through the vagina.

Calorie-wise, 1 teaspoonful of semen only has a few. The act of lovemaking, though, can burn off 100 calories easy.

Does what you eat affect the taste of your semen?

Some people seem to like the taste of semen, at least in the throes of passion, anyway. Others simply hate it. There are several different factors that can alter the flavor of your partner's semen. Diet is key. Just as the foods you eat can affect the smell of your breath, the foods you eat will affect the taste of your semen. Foods like asparagus, broccoli, spinach, coffee, and red meat can make semen rather sharp tasting. Conversely, celery, kiwi, pineapple, and watermelon will lend a milder taste to the ejaculate. Acidic fruits, like blueberries, cranberries, and plums, seem to lend a "pleasant," sugary flavor. Alkaline foods, like fish and some meats, impart a buttery flavor. Dairy products are said to make for a foul taste.

The more sperm there is in one's semen, the harsher it will be. If a man ejaculates several times in a couple days' time, there will be less sperm in his semen, and it will taste milder.

Other things that can make semen foul-tasting are smoking and drinking alcohol. A diabetic's sperm tends to taste sweeter.

Can a woman be allergic to semen?

Talk about being incompatible—some women are literally allergic to their mate. Well, to his semen anyway. Semen allergy is a rare condition that is often misdiagnosed as a yeast infection.

Women who suffer from semen allergies can experience localized burning, pain, and swelling in the vagina that can last for long periods of time. In its most common form, it affects the outer vagina, but it can irritate the inside as well. Sufferers may complain of the feeling of thousands of little needles being stuck into them simultaneously.

Other women may get a systemic response, including having trouble breathing, hives, and the swelling of soft tissues. In rare cases, they may pass out from anaphylaxis. Symptoms generally occur within 5 to 30 minutes.

So what's in semen that causes these reactions? It's the proteins in semen that trigger the woman's antibodies to kick into action in a systemic response. In a localized response the reaction may be more akin to what happens with poison ivy contact. This is similar to what happens with seasonal allergies.

It is also possible for a woman to have an oral reaction from taking semen into the mouth, although rarely. Semen that is swallowed is thought to be neutralized by the stomach's acids.

What's curious is that a woman may be allergic to one man's semen, but not another's. The most effective answer is for the man to wear a condom. This is a major problem for couples wanting to have a baby. Allergists can desensitize women to their partner's semen with injections similar to regular allergy shots. Proteins are separated out of the man's semen, and the woman undergoes a skin test to see which ones she is allergic to. Then the proteins she reacted to are injected into her every 10 to 15 minutes in gradually increasing concentrations, for several hours. Once the desensitizing is complete, she has the man's semen instilled into her vagina. If she shows no reaction, the treatment is deemed a success.

Other clinicians will instill increasing concentrations of semen directly into the vagina over time to achieve the same results. Either way, the treatments are costly and insurance companies don't cover them. Big surprise.

Do men have vaginas?

Guys do have some leftover female sex organs. All red-blooded, beer drinkin', truck drivin' men have what's known as a *vagina masculina*. In human embryos, there's something called the müllerian ducts. In a female, these develop into the uterus and fallopian tubes. In a male they shrivel up and become a little speck in the prostatic urethra, near the ejaculatory ducts.

Can men lactate?

Through the miracle of modern science many wondrous things are possible. One group of men actually did grow breasts and lactate, not that they wanted to. East Germans doctors, who were notorious for chemically altering their female athletes to become more masculine during the Cold War, also dabbled in feminizing a small segment of their male population, specifically convicted rapists.

Before the tearing down of the Berlin Wall, jailed rapists in the former East Germany were in for one weird and wild detention. To chill their overactive libidos, the rapists had implants inserted under their skin that released a slow, but steady supply of the female hormone estrogen. They soon began growing large fleshy breasts, complete with feminine nipples and areolae. And yes, some of these men did lactate!

What men can tie their penises into knots?

Aside from porn stars, the Karamojong people in northeastern Uganda love long penises. When a boy reaches puberty, they start tying circular stone disks onto the end of his unit, making it swing like a pendulum. Over time, the amount of weight is gradually increased, until weights of 20 pounds or more are reached! In the end, members 18 inches in length can be obtained. Sounds great, right? Well, the increase in length is offset by a decrease in girth. What they end up with is a long, thin floppy penis. As with the case of dangling labias, discussed in the last chapter, this can get in the way of everyday living. Hence, the Karamojong men tie their taffy-like dicks up in a knot, or even a double knot, to get them out of the way.

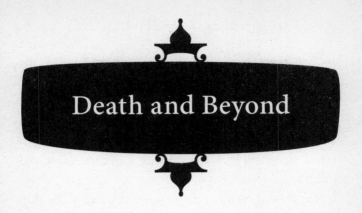

Death and Beyond

Death is our ultimate destiny—and it's not pretty. Any way you look at it, some mighty foul things happen to your body after you die. Humankind has always tried to come to grips with death's meaning and finality. Thus a multitude of rituals and practices have arisen, many of them quite bizarre and, yes, quite disgusting. Prepare yourself for a trip to the great (and gross) beyond.

What creatures eat your body when you die?

It's not pleasant, so brace yourself. The environment of the dead body changes rapidly over time and promotes a long succession of nasty animals that break down our remains.

The brain cells are the first to die, usually in 3 to 7 minutes. Skin cells can remain viable for up to 24 hours.

Almost immediately, bacteria swing into action. As

soon as rigor mortis sets in (within about 3 hours) the muscles become very acidic (with lactic acid). Anaerobic bacteria already in the body start to attack the intestines and other parts of the corpse. The body's own enzymes simultaneously begin breaking down tissue. The pancreas, for example, is loaded with digestive juices and quickly dissolves itself.

The rotting tissues release gases that cause the skin to blister and turn green. As the body swells, the tongue and eyes may bulge and fluids in the lungs will ooze from the mouth and nostrils.

After about 6 days in temperate climates, hydrogen sulfide and methane gases generate a nauseating stench. A corpse left unburied attracts a host of insects and animals. In the tropics, the process is much accelerated. A body can become a mass of wriggling maggots in 24 hours.

The stench of death is a signal for flies to move in. Although the flies cannot tolerate the acids found in the fluids leaking from the corpse, their larvae (maggots) can, and flies begin laying their eggs. Between the activities of the maggots and the bacteria, these acids are neutralized, making the now semiliquid cadaver attractive to blowflies, flesh flies, and houseflies.

The alkaline conditions created by the flies discourage beetles from feeding on the corpse, but they do enjoy eating the fly larvae. Parasitoid wasps are also present, laying their eggs in the fly larvae and pupae.

As time goes on, the corpse becomes too dry for maggots. Ham beetles, hide beetles, and carcass beetles now move in, devouring the dried-out flesh, cartilage, and ligaments. Finally, mites and moth larvae eat the hair, leaving only mankind's mortal residue—bones.

How are insects used to determine time of death?

Those of you who watch *CSI* or any other of the plethora of forensic science crime shows on TV today probably have a good idea. Insects colonize a corpse in a predictable order. The insects found in a corpse offer excellent clues as to time of death.

Temperature and humidity are two factors governing the timing of which insects will be found in a cadaver. As such, forensic scientists must consult weather bureau records to determine conditions present in the area of the corpse for the recent past. By collecting and raising the maggots of various flies present in the cadaver, they can determine how long the corpse has been lying around.

Where do they study rotting corpses?

The proper name for such a place is a body farm. There are two in the United States: one at the University of Tennessee-Knoxville and one at Western Carolina University.

The Federal Bureau of Investigation trains at the University of Tennessee facility, where agents learn how to dig up corpses and determine time of death. Medical examiners, law enforcement officials, and crime scene investigators all benefit from studying there. Located on a 3-acre wooded lot that is fenced off by razor wire, numerous bodies are scattered around the property, in various states of decay. They are treated in different ways to study environmental effects on body decomposition. Some are left in the open, others buried, others stuffed in the trunks of cars. The bodies are usually unclaimed cadavers from medical examiners, although 300 or so people have donated their bodies to the facility.

What causes rigor mortis?

As you must know, rigor mortis describes the stiffening of the muscles soon after death. It begins within 3 hours, reaching peak stiffness after 12 hours, and then gradually lessening until 72 hours after death. Why do the muscles react this way? Like everything else that happens to corpses, it's a matter of chemical reactions.

Muscles are composed of two types of fibers that have connections between them that lock and unlock as the muscle contracts and relaxes. Muscle contractions are controlled by the calcium ion levels found in the cells. When calcium ion levels increase, muscles contract. When they go down, muscles relax. Calcium levels are higher outside the muscle cells than within, so calcium ions tend to diffuse into the cell. Energy molecules are required to pump the ions back out across the cell membrane. These molecules depend on oxygen to function. Once a person stops breathing, oxygen levels go down, the calcium ion pumps quit, and the muscles go into severe contractions. They remain contracted until muscle proteins start to decay.

Why do embalmers massage corpses?

The first thing an embalmer does is to make sure the deceased is really deceased. You never know. Next the clothing and jewelry are removed and inventoried. For modesty's sake, a small cloth is usually placed over the genitals. The body is then disinfected and washed. Shaving and hairstyling are next, followed by bending, flexing, and massaging of the limbs to relieve rigor mortis. The eyes are kept closed with an eye cap and the mouth is held shut by means of suturing and adhesive. The tricky part is getting the mouth and facial expression to come out looking as natural and relaxed as possible. The next step is embalming.

Embalming fluid is designed for short-term preservation. It is composed of formaldehyde, ethanol, methanol, and other solvents. The embalmer uses a mechanical pump to inject the embalming fluid into the right carotid artery while blood is drained from the right jugular vein. The body is massaged to ensure uniform distribution of the embalming fluid.

If that weren't gross enough, the embalmer next must drain the fluids from the body cavities. They do so by making a cut 2 inches above and to the right of the belly button and inserting something called a trocar—a long, sharply pointed hollow metal tube. The trocar is attached to a pump via a hose. This gruesome device is inserted into the incision and moved about the chest and stomach cavities to puncture the organs and suck out their contents. Then the hose is detached from the pump and embalming fluid is added through it into the now-empty body cavities. Finally, a little plastic screw-in cap is placed in the incision to cork in the added fluids. Some preservatives may be injected just under the skin as needed.

On average, the grisly proceedings take 2 or 3 hours.

Do the dead *have* to be embalmed before a funeral?

Embalming may not be as essential as you have been lead to believe. It does not disinfect or preserve the body for long periods of time, regardless of what a funeral director may tell you. Embalming is done solely so the body looks lifelike for a short period and to make it easier for the mortician to work with. In some states it is not required by law before a funeral, if the condition of the body allows. A quick funeral, however, would be advisable.

Some states, like California, have no law on the books about how long you may keep a dead body at home, as there is no health concern involved. So, like a cheap wedding, you can also have an at-home funeral. If you choose to do so, check online for cheap coffin bargains.

Funeral homes generally mark up caskets. A $3,500 casket probably cost the funeral home only $700 wholesale.

In the Muslim tradition, embalming is strictly forbidden and the body should be buried within 24 hours, if possible. Traditional Jewish customs are similar.

Why didn't they embalm Pope John Paul II?

Maybe you heard that Pope John Paul II, who died in 2005, was not embalmed, but simply "prepared" for viewing. The Vatican has no formal doctrine on embalming. Pope John Paul II looks blotchy and bloated in photographs taken while he was lying in state. His body may have only been rubbed with myrrh, as was common in biblical times.

One twentieth-century pope who was embalmed, with horrific results, was Pope Pius XII. On his death, in 1958, a quack doctor convinced the Vatican to try a new embalming technique, which somehow actually sped up the decomposition of his body. His corpse turned black and his nose fell off as he was lying in state. So bad was the odor, that the Swiss guards watching over him had to take breaks every 15 minutes so as not to pass out.

Historically, the organs of deceased popes were removed to make the embalming more effective and long lasting. The relics of 22 popes, from Sixtus V, who died in 1590, to Leo VIII, who died in 1903, are kept in Rome's St. Anastasio and Vincent Church, near the

Trevi Fountain. The custom of removing organs was ended by Pope Pius X, who sat from 1903 to 1914.

Vladimir Lenin was kept submerged in a tank of fluids and was left out for public viewing for several decades after his death.

How are bodies made presentable for viewing?

As you might guess, cosmetics play a big role. Translucent makeup is applied to add depth to facial features. Heavier makeup is applied to hide any bruising or other discolorations. Men may have light pink lipstick applied to return a lifelike appearance. Light pink lighting can be used near the casket at the viewing to soften the deceased's complexion. Baby powder is used to lend a fresh fragrance to the corpse.

As far as clothing is concerned, it's up to the next of kin. Most bodies do not wear shoes because the feet usually have swollen.

How do they cremate someone?

There's a science to cremation. They don't just burn the body and collect the ashes. The chamber in which the body is incinerated is called the "retort" and is usually fueled by natural gas or propane. Temperatures can reach up to 1,800°F and are constantly monitored by an operator to ensure the most efficient burn. More jets of flame are directed at the torso because this is where most of the body mass is. Computers control much of the process. Once the retort reaches the optimal temperature, the casket is inserted quickly through a top-opening door.

Most of the body's soft tissue and fluids are vaporized and vented through an exhaust system to the outside air. In about 2 hours, the deceased is reduced mainly to ashes with some larger chunks of unburned bone mixed in. To achieve that nice fluffy powder the bereaved want to take home, the remains are swept out of the retort and pulverized in a cremulator—a rotating drum filled with steel ball bearings. What's left is 3 to 8 pounds of ashes, depending on the size of the body.

One thing about cremation you may not be aware of is that when they sweep the ashes out of the retort, they don't get every last bit. Consequently, there are ashes remaining from the preceding cremations that find their way into subsequent cremations. Aside from the remains of a stranger mixed in with your loved one's, there will also be various tiny incombustible things like dental fillings. (Larger pieces of metal, such as surgical screws and artificial joints, are removed with a magnet before pulverizing.)

One more thing about cremation—you can bring your own urn, if you like. Just check beforehand to make sure it's big enough.

Do they cremate the casket, too?

Most casket companies offer a line of combustible caskets for cremation. Sturdy cardboard box liners are also available that can be placed inside the fancy casket and removed for incineration, allowing the casket to be reused. (Why burn up a $5,000 box?) Casket rentals are also an option in many areas. After the funeral services, the deceased is put into a cheaper box for cremation.

Can you attend a cremation?

Should you so desire, you can watch the cremation of a loved one. However, if the dearly departed was morbidly obese, cremation is not an option because most retorts cannot handle bodies much above 400 pounds.

What historical figure drank the ashes of her husband?

One other bit of cremation trivia you may be amused by—the word *mausoleum* comes from the tomb of Mausolus, ruler of Caria (part of modern-day Turkey), who died in 353 BCE. His wife, Artesmia, who also happened to be his sister, had him cremated and kept his ashes on hand to drink with her wine from time to time. Before her death, she commissioned a tomb for him so splendid that it became one of the Seven Wonders of the Ancient World.

It's not only ancient nut jobs who might ingest human ashes. Keith Richards, of Rolling Stones fame, admitted in 2007 to snorting his father's ashes mixed with his cocaine.[1] After much play in the press, he later said he was only joking, but you never know.

What is "grave wax"?

Also known as "adipocere," grave wax is a whitish, crumbly, waxy substance that forms on fatty tissues of a cadaver, such as the abdomen, buttocks, breasts, and cheeks. It begins to form on corpses in a humid or wet environment after about a month and can remain for centuries if the corpse is not disturbed. The wax is a result of a chemical reaction of fats with water and hydrogen in the presence of bacterial enzymes, yielding fatty acid and soap.

One particularly hideous example of grave wax can be found in the Mütter Museum in Philadelphia. Known as the "Soap Woman," she is an obese woman who died in the 1800s and her body is almost entirely covered with grave wax.

Can a casket burp?

This rather unsettling phenomenon does indeed occur. As you know, when a body begins to decompose, all sorts of bacteria and enzymes are actively going about their business of breaking down tissue, producing noxious gases in the process that cause the body to bloat and the eyes to bulge out. Under the right circumstances, these gases may erupt. For this reason, the funeral industry designs casket seals that give way before enough pressure builds up inside to cause an explosion. (Now that would register a 10 on the gross meter!) Funeral business insiders euphemistically refer to the action of the seals giving way under pressure as "burping."

Legend has it that William the Conqueror of the Battle of Hastings fame was too big for his coffin when he died in 1087. Two soldiers are said to have jumped on him to squish his corpse into the casket, causing his gas-filled stomach to explode.

Were people inadvertently buried alive in the old days?

Mark Twain once quipped, "Rumors of my demise are greatly exaggerated." It's a funny line, but in Twain's day, the odd person *was* buried while still alive. This is one of the reasons people started holding wakes for the dead. By staying with the body right up until burial, family members could make sure their loved one was really dead. A festive gathering with lots of noisy people might "wake" the not-so-quite dead.

Before the days of modern medical science, a person in a coma might appear to be dead, and there are numerous documented cases of supposedly dead people who awoke. There's the story of Marjorie Elphinstone of Ardtannies, Scotland, who "died" and was buried in the early seventeenth century. Legend has it that grave robbers dug up her coffin soon after her burial and were shocked when she groaned and sat up. Supposedly, she climbed out of the casket and walked home to a stunned husband, whom she went on to outlive by 6 years.

Because of such nightmarish occurrences, people specified in their wills that certain precautions should be taken before they were buried, including pouring boiling water on them to see if they woke up, or stabbing them through the heart or decapitating them to make *sure* they were dead. Other folks requested a gun or poison be buried with them so they could kill themselves if they woke up 6 feet under. There was so much anecdotal evidence of people being buried alive that "hospitals for the dead" were set up in eighteenth-century Europe, where cadavers were laid out until they started to putrefy.

In the late 1880s, a guy named Count Karnice-Karnicki was so horrified when a young Belgian girl started screaming from within her casket as they started shoveling dirt on her, that he invented a coffin that would allow a buried person to signal people aboveground that they were still alive. It consisted of a hollow tube that extended to a box on the surface. A weighted ball attached to a chain in the box sat on the body's chest. If the body moved, the ball would shift, causing the chain to release a lid on the box, admitting air to the coffin and triggering a system of flags and bells. He received a patent for the casket in 1897.

There is still the odd report of people today reviving

after being pronounced dead by a coroner. In 1994, 86-year-old Mildred C. Clarke came back to life, 1½ hours after being zipped up in a body bag, in the morgue at the Albany Medical Hospital.[2] She had been found on her living room floor with no vital signs and stiff as a board. So you never know.

How are power saws used during an autopsy?

The word *autopsy* comes from the Greek *autopsia*, meaning "to see with one's own eyes." Maybe you know all about autopsies from watching those forensic medical shows on TV, maybe not. Autopsies aren't glamorous, and they aren't usually done by attractive people with beautifully coifed hair. There is at least one pathologist and one assistant, called a *diener* (German for "servant"; the practice of autopsy was largely developed in Germany).

And here are the steps in an average, run-of-the-mill autopsy:

- First the body is photographed and the outside is examined.
- The body is then cleaned, weighed, and measured.
- A rubber or plastic block is placed under the back so the head and arms fall backward and the chest is pushed outward.
- The torso is opened by making a Y-shaped incision starting from behind each ear, running down the

sides of the neck and meeting at the breastbone. A cut is then made across the collarbone from shoulder to shoulder and one long cut from the Adam's apple down to the pubic bone. There are slight variations in technique, depending on the pathologist and reason for the autopsy. Very little bleeding should occur because there is no cardiac function and gravity pulls the blood downward.

- The chest cavity is opened with an electric saw. Sometimes shears or scalpels are used instead because the saw creates a lot of dust as it rips through the bones. The sides of the rib cage are next sawed to allow the chest plate (sternum and attached ribs) to be lifted off in one piece, exposing the heart, lungs, and other organs in an undisturbed state.

- The pericardial sac is removed to expose the heart. Blood samples are taken from the pulmonary veins or inferior vena cava to check for bacteria. Blood, urine, bile, and even fluid from the eye may be sampled to look for medicines, street drugs, alcohol, or poisons. After examining the pulmonary artery for clots, the heart is cut out. The lungs and abdominal organs are next removed in a specific order after they've been examined in place. Sometimes pathologists will remove the organs as one block. This is usually the case with autopsies on infants.

- After removal, the organs are weighed, and tissue samples are taken. Blood vessels are opened, and the stomach and abdominal contents are examined.

By gauging the rate of digestion of the last meal, a rough time of death can be determined.

- The body block under the back is now placed under the head. A cut is made from behind one ear, up over the top of the head, and down to the other ear. The scalp is pulled away from the skull, with one large flap of skin flopped over the face and the other over the back of the neck. The electric saw is then used to cut a cap out of the skull, much as you would do to a jack-o'-lantern. After examining the brain, the spinal cord is severed and is removed. If it is to be saved, the brain is stored in a container of formalin to preserve it and make it firmer for later examination.

After the autopsy procedure, the body must be reassembled, with the possibility of a viewing and funeral in mind. The internal organs are either poured back into the chest cavity or incinerated. Then the chest and head are sewn back together with a big needle and thread, and the body is washed. Strategic positioning of the pillow in the casket will hide any marks from the brain's removal. If it is properly done, there will be no sign that an autopsy has been performed when the body is displayed for a funeral.

The fluid and tissue samples are examined at a later time, and a final report is ready in about a month. Sample slides and tissue are kept indefinitely so that the findings can be reviewed at a future date, if needed.

Are all autopsies the same?

There are two types of autopsies: clinical and forensic. A clinical autopsy is done to determine the medical cause of death in cases of unknown or undetermined death. A forensic autopsy is performed when it is suspected that foul play may have been involved. A forensic autopsy will place the death into one of five categories—natural, accidental, homicide, suicide, or undetermined.

The government can order an autopsy during a criminal investigation if there is some public health concern such as suspicion of a contagious disease or if someone dies without an attending doctor.

An autopsy can also be requested by the family of the deceased, if they wish to know more about the cause of death. These autopsies are generally done for free. In about one in four autopsies, the physician will find some major disease present that was not known about in life.[3] Private autopsies can also be performed in the funeral home. It doesn't matter if the body has been embalmed yet or not.

What people mummified their dead and gave the tongues to their relatives?

It's always nice to have something to remember the dearly departed by. How about keeping his or her tongue, or palms, or soles of the feet? This was the practice of the people of the Melanesian Islands.

When a loved one died, his or her body was left out in the sun for a few days, before being stuck in a canoe and sailed out to sea. Next, the skin was peeled off and the internal organs were removed and replaced with palm pith. The corpse was then returned to land, where it was hung up to dry on a wooden frame. Holes were made in the knees, elbows, and hands to let the bodily fluids drain out. Finally, the tongue, palms, and soles of the feet were cut off and given to the next of kin.

Once the mummy was fully dried out, it was decorated with seashells and grass and painted with red ocher. This ornate corpse was then placed on a pole in the home of the surviving spouse, where, over time, it fell apart, leaving just the head, and a fond memory.

What people keep the head of the deceased for a drinking cup?

Some of the Aboriginal peoples of Australia liked to dry mummify their dead. They removed the body fat, mixed it with red ocher, and painted the body with it. Next, they sewed shut the mouth, eyes, ears, and other body holes lower down, and put the corpse up on a platform above a fire to be smoked like a ham.

For 10 days, mourners would stand around the body as it was being smoked, not saying a word. A couple of guards would wave emu feathers or branches to keep flies off the cadaver. After several weeks of smoking, the corpse was hung in a tree or put on another platform, and the skull given to the family to use as a drinking vessel.

What people mummified themselves?

Beginning around 1000 BCE, Buddhist priests in Japan began trying to turn themselves into mummies—while they were still living. How does one mummify oneself? you may ask. It isn't easy. For a period of 3 years, the priests would go on a very strict diet, eating only tree bark and nuts, essentially starving themselves and becoming quite anorexic. As they began to lose weight, they would place lots of candles all around themselves, to dry out the skin from the candles' heat. By the time the priest died from starvation, he was close to being a mummy. To complete the mummification process, his body would be placed in an underground tomb for 3 more years and then surrounded by candles again to finish drying him out.

Apparently, malnutrition caused the internal organs and muscles to shrink and dry out, thus destroying bacteria and preserving the corpse.

Some 19 of these mummified priests still exist today. They are kept in Buddhist monasteries around the island of Honshu, Japan. There used to be hundreds of such mummies in China as well; but during the Cultural

Revolution, when the Chinese leaders ordered their desecration, the Buddhists had them cremated.

What religion leaves their dead out for vultures?

Maybe you've heard of the Zoroastrians. Zoroastrianism is based on the teachings of the Bronze Age Persian prophet Zoroaster (Zarathustra) and recognizes Ahura Mazda as its divine authority. At one time, Zoroastrianism was the main religion of large areas of central and western Asia. Today, its adherents number about 200,000, primarily in India and Iran.

Zoroastrians believe that after death, the soul departs the body, leaving an empty shell. Corpses, and hair and nail clippings, are thought to be impure. They hold fire to be a symbol of God's spirit, so burning "unclean" corpses would be a mortal sin. Burying the dead would likewise contaminate the earth. What to do? Just let the corpses rot.

Dead bodies cannot be touched by anyone except special corpse bearers who live outside of the community. They bathe the body in special urine from a white bull as an aid to purification, and wrap it in linen. Traditionally, the dead are then placed on a raised open stone structure called a *Dakhma*, or Tower of Silence, and left there to be eaten by vultures and eroded by the elements. Bodies are arranged in three rings, with the men on the outside, women next, and children in the center. After about a year, the remaining bones, which have been bleached by the sun, are put into pits and eventually washed out to sea.

Towers of Silence have been banned in Iran, but are used by the 82,000 members of the Parsi sect in India, most of whom live in Mumbai. One modern-day problem with this practice is that there is a shortage of meat-eating birds left in India. Millions of them have died from eating cow carcasses contaminated with painkillers given to sick cattle. As a result, some bodies are not fully stripped of their flesh. Concerned Parsis are considering a breeding program for vultures. Solar concentrators have also recently been employed to speed decomposition along.

Objections to the practice are being raised by many of Mumbai's 16 million other residents. It seems that with three or four Parsi dying every day, the stench from the rotting piles of corpses has become overwhelming.

Where can you go to learn more about funerals?

Are you fascinated by funerals and funeral memorabilia? Then check out the Museum of Funeral Customs in Springfield, Illinois. For a mere $4 (kids $2!) you can see such displays as a re-created 1920s embalming room, a re-created 1870 funeral home, postmortem photographs, coffins and caskets from throughout the ages, and a replica of Lincoln's casket. Don't forget to stop by the gift shop to pick up some chocolate candy coffins, a horse-drawn-hearse-emblazoned Christmas ornament, or a book on embalming.

If you live closer to Houston, Texas, check out the National Museum of Funeral History instead. It is a little pricier at $6 a head. Corpses admitted for free.

Spain also has a quite interesting museum. Barcelona's Municipal Funeral Services building houses one of the world's finest collections of funeral carriages and hearses. The Museum of Funeral Carriages occupies the basement under the city morgue. (How fitting.) It's terrifying, and best of all, it's free.

Where do they dig up dead relatives' bones for parades?

In Madagascar there is a strange practice called *famadihana,* in which families dig up the bones of their buried relatives and march them around the village. The bones are then wrapped in a new shroud and reburied. Now for the really strange and gross part. They give the old burial shrouds to newlywed couples to cover their connubial bed. (How erotic.)

How long does the human head remain conscious after decapitation?

Beheading today is rather rare, except in a few countries, like Saudi Arabia, Qatar, and Yemen, that still permit it. Years ago, beheading was common, especially in the reign of Henry VIII in England and during the French Revolution.

During the French Reign of Terror, from September 1793 to July 1794, it has been estimated that between 18,000 and 40,000 people were executed, most with the guillotine. So many heads were rolling that the executioners became very familiar with the immediate effects on the head after being removed from the neck. Some said that they spoke to the bodiless heads within seconds of beheading and were able to elicit a response.

It has been suggested that the human head remains conscious for 15 to 20 seconds after decapitation, although solid medical evidence is lacking. Deprivation of oxygen to the brain for any longer results in loss of consciousness. Studies in rats show a cessation of electrical activity in the brain 30 seconds after decapitation, indicating brain death.

What famous person's wife carried his head around for 29 years?

Some bereaved folks just can't seem to let go of the dearly departed. Sir Walter Raleigh's wife had his noggin embalmed after he was beheaded in 1618. She carried it with her for the next 29 years.

Mary Shelley was just as attached to her husband, poet Percy Bysshe. The famed author of *Frankenstein* kept her husband's heart when his fish-eaten corpse washed up on the beach after he drowned in 1822.

One woman who was forced to keep a body part of her lover, against her will, was Catherine, wife of Peter the Great. Peter, who was quite a philanderer himself, had Catherine's lover, William Mons, beheaded and made her keep the head in a jar of alcohol next to her bed as a reminder of her infidelity.

One other famous person who had a body part preserved was Albert Einstein. When he died in 1955, his body was cremated. But his brain was retained by Princeton Hospital pathologist Thomas S. Harvey, who kept it in two mason jars in his home.

What king had the corpse of his mistress exhumed to crown her queen? (and other dead trivia)

- In 1355, King Pedro of Portugal had the corpse of his dead mistress exhumed and crowned queen at his coronation. Subjects had to kneel and kiss her decomposed hand.
- Hair and nails don't grow after death. It just appears that way since the body starts to shrink.
- Jerome Rodale, organic food health guru and founder of Rodale Press, died on *The Dick Cavett Show,* the day after boasting he was going to live to be 100. His head slumped to his chest, and Cavett

asked him, "Are we boring you, Mr. Rodale?" It was no gag. The tape of the show, complete with medics rushing onto the stage, was never aired. He was 72 at the time.

What culture eats their dead?

The Fore tribe of Papua, New Guinea, had some nasty experiences when they began eating their dead at mortuary rituals. They started devouring their dead in the late 1800s and persisted in doing so until Western missionaries stamped out the practice in the 1950s. According to oral tradition, when a Fore tribal member died, the maternal relatives would dismember the body. Once rotting began, they would cut off the feet and arms, remove the muscles from the limbs, and take out the internal organs and brain.

The men at these ceremonies ate the best meat, the muscles, while women and children ate the brains and intestines. This gruesome meal had a rather unfortunate side effect. The women and children, predominantly, contracted the prion disease kuru (which is related to mad cow disease) from eating infected brains.

Also known as "laughing sickness," the second stage of kuru made one laugh uncontrollably. Victims became paralyzed and their brains started to resemble Swiss cheese, with holes throughout. About 200 Fore died annually from the disease between 1920 and 1960.

Certain Amazon tribes also had a unique way to honor the dead. They would wrap them up in their hammock and cook them whole in a big clay pot (not the big metal cauldron like you see in the cartoons). Once all the meat was cooked off, the bones were washed, powdered, and sprinkled in their corn soup. (Does Campbell's know about this?)

What peoples practiced cannibalism?

Cannibalism is probably the most universal human taboo, in modern times, anyway. There is, however, evidence of cannibalism among our prehistoric ancestors. Cannibalism is mentioned in the Bible (2 Kings 6:25–30). In this text, during the famine and siege of Samaria, two women agree to kill their children and eat them. The first woman boiled her son, and they ate him. Later, when it was time for the second woman to boil her son, he had conveniently disappeared (she reneged).

The Aztecs were notorious cannibals. They cooked up a corn-man dish called *tlacatlaoll*. The Egyptians resorted to the practice when the Nile failed to flood for several years. During the First Crusade, the Crusaders were forced to eat the enemy dead due to lack of food. The settlers at Jamestown are also believed to have eaten their dead.

The islands of Fiji had a long history of cannibalism. The most prolific cannibal of all time (the most prolific we know about, that is) was the nineteenth-century Fiji chief Ratu Udre Udre, who kept a stone record of the 872 to 999 people he had eaten. It is placed by his tomb. His son reported that the grisly chief would eat every part of his victims, saving what he couldn't finish in one sitting for later meals. Fijians believed that one gained the spiritual strength of one's foes by eating their flesh. The defeated enemies were first cooked in pit ovens. Special four-pronged forks were used for the macabre meals. It was considered bad form for the meat to touch one's lips. (Even cannibals had their rules of etiquette!)

With their conversion to Christianity, cannibalism died out among the Fijians. The last occurrence of cannibalism there took place in 1867, when a chief devoured a Wesleyan Methodist missionary who had inadvertently touched his head, a definite no-no—even today. In 2003, the Fiji islanders descended from the chief who ate the missionary, publicly apologized to his descendants, believing that this would lift a curse they felt was bringing them bad luck.

Today, cannibalism is pretty much dead everywhere, except for the Korowai tribe of southeastern Papua, New Guinea, and a few crazy psycho killers. Supposedly, the Korowai punish those convicted of secret witchcraft by torturing them and then eating their brain while it is still warm.

The most infamous case of recent cannibalism happened in 1979 when the Uruguay rugby team's plane crashed high in the Andes. The survivors were not rescued for 70 days, during which time they were compelled to eat the dead. Some of their members wandered far away from the wreckage to die to avoid suffering such a postmortem fate.

What is self-cannibalism?

As the word suggests, self-cannibalism, also known as "autophagy," is the eating of one's self. Obviously, as a survival technique this strategy can't be taken too far. Mice have been known to eat their own tails when starving. The short-tailed cricket can eat its own wings in a pinch. Octopi affected by a virus or bacteria may chew on their tentacles to relieve pain or itching, and some animals have chewed off a limb when caught in a trap.

Some people engage in autophagy. Technically speaking, if you eat your boogers, pick a scab and eat it, or chew your fingernails, this is self-cannibalism. Some mentally unstable people will peel off bits of their skin and eat it.

Do people have white meat and dark meat?

Sure, chickens and turkeys have white meat and dark meat, but what about people? Yes, in humans, just as in birds, the muscles that do a lot of work contain darker meat. Dark meat is made up of muscles with fibers that are known as type 2, or slow-twitch. These are endurance muscles that are used for extended periods of time and thus need more oxygen than type 1, or fast-twitch muscles, which are used only for short bursts of activity.

Myoglobin is the richly pigmented protein that stores

oxygen in the muscles. Slow-twitch muscles contain more myoglobin and mitochondria than do fast-twitch muscles. Hence, the redder, darker meat. As in chickens, our endurance muscles—the calves and thighs—are dark meat.

OK, you are dying to know, right? Human flesh is said to taste just like pork. And you thought it was going to be chicken.

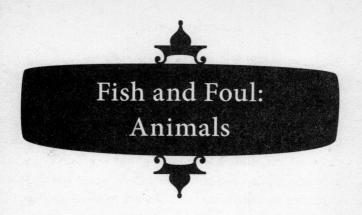

Fish and Foul: Animals

We humans consider ourselves quite cultured and refined. Throughout the course of our history, we have become almost completely distanced from any aspect of life that we find disgusting. We answer "the call of nature" in special places, wear clothing to protect and hide our bodies, and are obsessed with hygiene and manners (well, most of us are, anyway). Animals have no such concerns. Theirs is a wild and often foul existence (anthropomorphically speaking). To find out just how foul, read on.

Do fish communicate by farting?

Biologists have linked a mysterious underwater farting sound to bubbles that come out of a herring's anus. (Who pays for this research?) Ben Wilson, a research associate with the Fisheries Centre at the University of

British Columbia, says, "It sounds just like a high-pitched raspberry."[1] Apparently, the fish use the high-frequency farts for communication. This is a new phenomenon in marine biology, so the researchers had to come up with a fancy term for it—fast repetitive tick (FRT). (Calling it "fish farting" just won't do when it comes time to request more federal grant money.) Extensive testing has led the biologists to speculate that FRT is used by the herring to keep the school intact after dark. That's good to know. Now on to other business.

What fish has the grossest form of reproduction?

There are a couple of very curious characteristics of the deep-water anglerfish (order Lophiiformes). For starters, they derive their name from the fact that they really are anglers—that is, they fish for their meals. Anglers have a rod-like appendage with an irregular bit of flesh on the end that hangs down in front of their mouth. This rod is wiggled about to attract the interest of other fish. When one touches the rod, the anglerfish swallows it. Pretty neat. Their method of reproduction, however, is pretty gross.

The male anglerfish is born with no digestive system. He must quickly find a female or else he will die. Upon finding a female, the male bites into her flank and releases an enzyme that dissolves the flesh in his mouth and the flesh where he bit her, allowing for a fusion of the two fish down to the blood vessel level. He then withers away, becoming essentially nothing more than a sac of gonads ready to release sperm when the female releases her eggs. Hormones in her blood flow tell the gonads when to do so.

Such a system of sexual dimorphism ensures that the female's eggs will always be fertilized in a deep-sea environment where males may be hard to come by when the time is right.

Can turtles breathe through their butts?

Of course they can. Can't you? Turtles are one of the only animals (sea cucumbers and dragonfly nymphs are some others) that can "breathe" through their anus. They suck water into their cloaca (the tube that they use to pass feces, urine, and sexual fluids) and into two special sacs. These pockets are lined with blood vessels that can absorb oxygen from the water they contain. Some turtles can get 70 percent of their oxygen by butt breathing. This ability comes in quite handy when the turtles sleep underwater.

How do porcupines make love?

"Very carefully!" is the answer to this old joke. This is indeed the case. Porcupine sex is a delicate affair, to put it mildly. After the male becomes aroused, he stands on his hind legs, several feet away from the object of his desire and proceeds to urinate on her. This golden shower is not well received by the female, who snaps and growls at him. The male then approaches her, usually on three legs, stroking his penis with the fourth. Now comes the tricky part of the courtship. The female must fold down *all* of her rear quills. If everything goes well, he mounts her from the rear and penetration will follow. At times, young, inexperienced female porcupines don't fold down all their quills, or forget to move their barbed tail out of the way. This tends to complicate matters and can be a bit of a pain for the male.

Why do skunks stink?

The word *skunk* comes from the Algonquian word *seganku*, or *segonku*, meaning "one who squirts." The genus name of the common striped skunk is *Mephitis*, which means "stench" or "reek." Of course, skunks' smell is a defensive tactic. Once squirted, neither man nor beast will likely mess with a skunk again (except maybe your dopey dog). But what makes that God-awful stench?

Skunks have a scent gland on either side of their anus. This is where the oily, noxious fluid of sulfur-containing chemicals is squirted from. It may be one of the most powerful and obnoxious odors in the animal kingdom. Even if you've never seen a skunk up close, you know its smell. The odor can linger for days, especially if one gets squashed on the roadside, and can be detected for up to a mile away. Muscles next to the scent glands enable the skunk to shoot its foul spray 10 feet with great accuracy. If it hits you in the eyes, it can cause temporary blindness.

You really have to annoy a skunk to get sprayed though. Skunks have only five or six good blasts worth of chemical stored up, and it takes about 10 days to replenish it, so they don't want to waste their spray. You'll know what's coming before a skunk sprays because it will go through an elaborate routine of foot stomping, hissing, teeth chattering, and tail raising before firing. If you see this display, run for the hills.

Most predators avoid the skunk. Its only real enemy is the great horned owl, whose olfactory senses are so poor that the stink doesn't bother it.

What male animal "does it" until he dies from exhaustion?

Maybe the horniest creature in the animal kingdom is the male brown antechinus, an Australian mouse-size marsupial. They are carnivorous and belong to the same family as the Tasmanian devil. They also like to do it like crazy. When 11 months old, the males begin an intense 2-week breeding frenzy in order to father as many offspring as possible. Each male will copulate for about 6 hours at a time with as many females as possible until he dies from sheer exhaustion at the end of the mating season. (Not a bad way to go.)

Why do vultures have a bald head?

There are two main groups of vulture—Old World vultures and New World vultures. Old World vultures find their dinner exclusively by means of sight, but New World vultures also use the sense of smell. It's the mercaptan (sulfur-containing) gas made by rotting flesh that attracts them.

Circling vultures don't necessarily mean there is something dead below. They also circle to gain altitude, or just to have a little fun. The reason they don't just swoop down on fresh carrion and dig in is that they tend to have weak beaks. It's much easier for them to rip the guts out of a slightly decayed animal. They may peck out the eyes first, but they prefer the intestines.

Most vultures have a bald head. This is not a fashion statement but is for purely hygienic reasons. As vultures are always sticking their heads into rotting carcasses, they would quickly become a disgusting bloody mess if their heads were covered with feathers. A bald head makes for easier cleaning up in any nearby body of water.

Do vultures vomit in self-defense?

Vultures will eat until they almost literally burst. After a good meal they are so full that they may not be able to fly. In a pinch, they can regurgitate some of their dinner and beat a hasty retreat. They also vomit in self-defense. If threatened, they will puke up a hunk of stinking half-digested meat to deter predators from entering their nests. They can also vomit in the face of their foes, which will sting their eyes and drive them off.

As you would think, vultures have cast-iron stomachs. They can eat rotting meat containing anthrax, botulism, or cholera with no ill effects.

Turkey vultures also like to urinate on their own legs. Why? Because vultures cannot sweat in hot weather like we can, the evaporating pee has a cooling effect. Also, their pee has strong acids that help kill any bacteria on their feet that they picked up from stepping in their last meal.

What bird uses its poop as a weapon?

The European fieldfare is a bird with a quite unique defense mechanism. These birds are thrushes that defecate en masse on their predator enemies, such as the raven, in defense of their nests. The aerial bombardment destroys the oils on the feathers of their foes, ruining its waterproofing qualities. This may prove detrimental or fatal to the targeted birds. The fieldfare's scientific name is appropriately enough *Turdus pilaris*.

What other birds use vomit as a weapon?

Being pooped on is no picnic; neither is being vomited on. Fulmars and petrels, both seabirds, use regurgitation to defend their nest sites. The chicks will shoot regurgitated fish oil in the face on an attacking predator. Their projectile vomit can travel up to 20 feet. The yellowish stomach oils will adhere to the aggressor's feathers or fur, causing them to mat down. This destroys their insulating qualities and seabirds can drown when their matted feathers become waterlogged.

Birds aren't the only creatures that puke in self-defense. Distressed camels will also bring up the contents of their stomachs, along with saliva, and project it out at whatever is annoying them. This noxious stream is meant to surprise and distract. No doubt it does both.

What animals shoot blood out of their eyes?

Sounds like something from a horror movie or a weird Japanese cartoon, but it's actually the horned toad, a fairly common pet. Not really a toad, it's technically a horned lizard (*Phrynosoma*). There are 14 species of horned lizards in North America, 8 of them in the United States, commonly in Texas. These guys have spines on their backs and horns on their heads. They look sort of like a mini dinosaur.

Horned toads are quite docile, preferring to hide if approached by a predator. If provoked, they will try to run away. If this doesn't work, they puff up their bodies to look bigger and more fearsome. Finally, as a last resort, there are 4 species that can shoot blood from the corners of their eyes for a distance of 3 feet.

How can a creature shoot blood from its eyes? They are able to increase the blood pressure in their head to such a point that the blood vessels in the eyelids rupture, causing the blood to squirt from their tear ducts. Not only will this confuse a predator but many find the blood very nasty tasting. Birds, however, don't seem to mind.

What animal eats its own poop?

What animal is cuter and more adorable than a bunny rabbit? Rabbits and hares (along with pikas) are lagomorphs. They all have short tails and large hind feet with smaller forefeet. They are also all herbivores and engage in coprophagy, or the eating of their own feces.

Rabbits make two kinds of droppings, depending on the time of day. When they are active, rabbits make the familiar hard pellets you find in your yard. When they retire to their burrows to rest, they begin making soft, gooey, black, partially digested pellets that they eat as soon as they are passed. Rabbits reingest up to 82 percent of their feces. They swallow these soft pellets whole. The pellets are composed of partially digested plant material and bacteria, wrapped in a mucous membrane. The tough membrane keeps the pellets intact for at least 6 hours after reingestion, giving the bacteria more time to break down the vegetative matter, before it is redigested in a special part of the stomach. These soft pellets are an important source of nutrition.

Surprised? Don't you remember the Looney Tunes episode in which Bugs ate his own droppings? (Just kidding, that was Porky.)

What animals eat their parents' droppings?

The young of many species need particular bacteria in their guts to properly digest their food. One such example is the iguana (*Iguana iguana*). The only way for them to acquire these bacteria is from the droppings of adult iguanas who already possess the required microbes. This fact was discovered when young iguanas bred in captivity died in spite of receiving a proper diet.

Immature termites and cockroaches also eat the poop of adults to round out their digestive flora.

Can dead whales explode?

In 2004, a gross story from Taiwan made headlines. Marine biologists were moving a 56-foot-long whale carcass on a flatbed truck through the city of Tainan, on its way to the National Cheng Kung University, for a necropsy. They didn't get it there in time. The internal gases of the whale built up so much pressure that the 60-ton sperm whale exploded on a downtown street, showering cars, shops, and pedestrians with blood, blubber, and entrails. Talk about a mess!

What was left of the whale was then sent to a nature preserve instead of the university, where it caused another stir. It seems the beast had a formidable five-foot-long penis that fascinated local men. More than 100 showed up to gawk at the prodigious pecker.

A more infamous whale explosion took place in Florence, Oregon, on November 12, 1970. What was crazy about this one was that the 7-ton whale was blown up intentionally on the beach by the Oregon Highway Department. Not wanting the carcass to rot on the sand, someone at the department had the brilliant idea to pack the whale with a half a ton of dynamite and blow it to bits for seagulls and other scavengers to feast on. The whale was duly detonated and, predictably, pieces of gore went flying everywhere. All the curiosity seekers on the beach were drenched with blood and guts, and blubber flew up to ¼ mile away. One washing machine–size chunk smashed a parked car. Apparently, none of the geniuses at the department thought about just towing the dead whale out to sea.

Why do cows chew their cud?

Cud? What is this stuff anyway? And why do cows like to chew it? Perhaps you know that cows have four stomachs instead of just one. Why do they need four stomachs? Because they are ruminants, like goats, deer, buffaloes, giraffes, et al. Each stomach does a different part of the digestion process using different enzymes.

When a cow grabs a mouthful of grass, she just gives it a quick chew and swallows it, sending it to the first stomach—the rumen. Here the cellulose of the grass begins to break down, making the grass softer. She regurgitates the grass from the rumen back into her mouth for some more chewing. Then it's swallowed again into the second stomach—the reticulum—where it's broken down even more. From here it's off to stomach three—the omasum—where all the water is removed from the grassy goo. The final steps of digestion take place in stomach four—the abomasums—where an enzyme called rennet is made. (Rennet, obtained from the stomachs of slaughtered calves, is used to curdle the milk in the cheese-making process.)

What is the most hideous mammal?

This is a judgment call, but if you have ever seen a naked mole rat (*Heterocephalus glaber*) you will probably agree. They are mammals, but just barely. Naked mole rats are burrowing rodents from the grasslands of East Africa—Kenya, Somalia, and southern Ethiopia. They live an underground existence in extensive tunnel systems they dig with their large, protruding teeth.

They are pretty small, measuring 8 to 10 centimeters in length. Their eyes are just tiny slits, and their eyesight is very poor, which is OK because they live in total darkness. What makes them particularly hideous is their total lack of hair, except inside their mouths. Naked mole rats are the only totally hairless mammals. They are covered in folds of very wrinkled, pink or yellow skin, somewhat resembling a newborn gerbil. When they are born, their skin is so transparent that you can see right inside them.

They are also unique in that they have no fat layer, no sweat glands, and their skin can feel no pain. Although considered mammals, naked mole rats are virtually cold-blooded. They cannot regulate their body temperature at all and rely on an environment with a constant temperature to stay warm. But what really sets them apart from other mammals is the fact that they live a eusocial lifestyle, much like ants, bees, and termites.

Like the ants, naked mole rats live together in large underground colonies of 80 or more. Only one female—the queen, who is twice the size of the others—and one to three males are allowed to reproduce. The rest are workers, divided into groups with specific tasks, such as diggers or soldiers.

The breeding males will service the queen for many years. A queen can live for up to 18 years; and during this time, she is extremely hostile to other females. Her urine contains hormones that keep the ladies-in-waiting sterile until she dies. When the queen does finally croak, the other females engage in a violent struggle to ascend to the throne.

Mole rats live off tubers they find during their mining

operations. During lean times they will eat their own droppings, which they deposit in special "bathroom" chambers.

What tropical fish will burrow into your privates?

There's a fish that swims in the Amazon and Orinoco Rivers of South America that is even more feared by the local population than the infamous piranha. It's called the toothpick or candirú fish (*Vandellia cirrhosa*) and is a member of the catfish family. Why would a member of the catfish family be more fearsome than the piranha? For one rather nasty habit it has.

Known as the "vampire fish of Brazil," this little devil is 1 to 2 inches in length, as thin as a toothpick, and nearly translucent in the water, so it's almost impossible to see. It makes its living as a parasite, entering the gill slits of other fish, inserting a spine to hold itself in place, and feeding on the blood of its victims. What's so scary about that? Well, it's attracted to blood and urine. You know what this means. Nude bathers who pee in the water are asking for trouble. The toothpick fish will home in on the source and do its thing. It will enter your anus, vagina, or penis just as readily as some fish's gill slit.

This scaly vampire can burrow deep into your urethra (pee tube), fasten its barb, and start sucking your blood out of the most sensitive of places. The only way to extract it is through surgery and there probably aren't too many surgeons handy while you're bathing in the Orinoco. Thus the natives have a traditional cure to kill and dissolve the beast, which involves putting two plants (or their extracts, in the case of the penis) into the affected orifice. The only problem is that most people die of shock from infection before this works. (If they put the little guys in your local pool, they wouldn't have to worry about kids relieving themselves in the water anymore!)

What fish exudes slime as a self-defense?

Have you ever heard of hagfish (*Myxine glutinosa*)? They look more like eels than fish and have been dubbed by the scientific press as the most disgusting creatures in the seas.[2] Their claim to that title rests in the fact that they exude copious amounts of slime. When attacked or threatened, hagfish produce a thick mucus that makes them extremely slippery and may confuse or choke predators. By tying themselves in an overhand knot that works its way from the head to the tail, they can slip from the jaws of another fish. Fishermen have found that hagfish can make enough slime to fill a bucket in just 2 hours' time.

As if the slime thing weren't gross enough, hagfish also have a disgusting method of eating. They enter the body orifices of other fish, living or dead, through the mouth, gills, or anus, and eat their insides. This isn't exactly the kind of fish you want to keep in your saltwater aquarium at home.

What eel will bite you and never let go?

That would be the moray. Although there are many nasty eels—the electric and the lamprey (which isn't really an eel)—the moray is in a class by itself. The moray eel is a bit of a recluse. They hide in cracks and crevices in the ocean's reefs, only occasionally poking their heads out. They really want nothing to do with people whatsoever. Divers, on the other hand, like to go looking for the eel, so they can feed them by hand.

In aquarium situations, morays get used to their human feeders and look forward to their visits. In the wild, a spooked eel can become quite vicious. Once it sinks its teeth into you, it will never let go. So how do you get it off? If still in the water, you can try to lure it away with a dead fish. Because this is not usually practicable, the best way is to just cut its head off and head to the hospital ASAP.

By the by, the lamprey eel has no jaws. Its sucker-like mouth attaches to the side of a fish with rows of teeth that burrow through the flesh, enabling the eel to suck out body fluids, killing the fish.

What other animal will bite into you and not let go?

Like the moray eel, the desert-dwelling Gila monster (*Heloderma suspectum*) of the American Southwest has a fearsome bite. They also will sink their teeth into you and refuse to let go. The Gila monster will chomp down ½ inch into your flesh with a vise-like grip and hang on so its venom can enter the wound. They may even chew or tear at the flesh to let the poison penetrate farther.

Their venom probably won't kill you, but you will experience a burning pain, followed by swelling, possible bleeding, nausea, vomiting, thirst, and faintness. Hopefully, you can remove the critter before you are incapacitated, which ain't easy. Experts recommend placing a stick between the bite and the back of the lizard's mouth and pushing against the rear of the jaw. If this doesn't work, try applying a flame under the jaw or immerse it in water if any is handy. Only as a last resort should you grasp the lizard by the tail and remove it with a single jerk. In some cases, not even pliers can pry the animal loose.

Do vampire bats really drink blood?

Bats creep a lot of people out. Some folks believe they can somehow get stuck in your hair and will need to be cut out. Others, not many, think they are cute little mice with wings. Hollywood has contributed to the bad rap bats seem to have. Try to think of a movie in which bats have been portrayed in a positive light. Can't? All that comes to mind are vampires and icky caves.

Of the 850 or so bat species, only 3 are known to drink blood, and fortunately usually not human blood.

The 3 vampire bat species are the common vampire bat (*Desmodus rotundus*), which drinks the blood of mammals; the hairy-legged vampire bat (*Diphylla ecaudata*), which likes bird blood; and the white-winged vampire bat (*Diaemus youngi*), which also fancies bird blood. They live in Central and South America.

Unlike in the movies, in which they dive at your throat, real vampire bats are more sneaky. The common vampire bat's main prey is likely to be a cow, not a person. They stealthily approach their prey on the ground and climb up the leg, just above the hoof, or crawl behind the ear. Then they use their razor-sharp teeth to cut away the animal's fur and make a 7-millimeter-long long by 8-millimeter-deep cut in the flesh. Contrary to popular fiction, bats do not suck blood, they lick it up. An anticoagulant in the bat's saliva called draculin, appropriately enough, keeps the blood flowing.

The common vampire bat has special infrared sensors on its nose that can find where an animal's blood flows close to the skin. This guarantees striking blood every time. These bats are also able to detect the breathing sounds of sleeping animals; this makes choosing a place for dinner much easier.

Bats are very weight conscious. Not for shallow cosmetic reasons but because if they get too heavy it's hard to fly. Therefore, the whole time they are drinking in fresh blood at the front end, they are peeing on their host out the back end. Bats have the amazing ability to begin to digest their blood meal and eliminate its waste products in about 2 minutes. This is really important because the average bat weighs about 40 grams and can drink 20 grams of blood in a typical 20-minute feeding.

Far from being bloodthirsty savages, bats are very social, living in colonies that number in the millions. They also watch out for each other. If one bat is too ill or feeble to fly out for an evening meal, one of his comrades will bring him back a blood meal that he pukes up for his friend to lick out of his mouth.

One other bit of bat trivia: The reason they hang upside down is because their little legs are too weak to support them standing upright.

What bugs are used to strip skeletons?

Want to see bones, lots of bones? Head to a museum. They seem to love them. But how do they get bones for display? Say they collect a dead rhino, or some other creature. How do they get rid of all the flesh and end up with nice clean bones? There are several methods, but using beetles is the best.

A common beetle often found on roadkill is the dermestid, or carpet beetle. Museums collect them from the local population (rotting carcasses). They are easily raised in captivity, can't fly away when the temperature is below 80°F, and eat large quantities of flesh.

Museum workers remove the hides and organs from animal specimens. They are then placed in a box with these bugs and moistened paper towels. Small specimens may be stripped clean in one night. Others may require several days. After the beetles have done their work, museum workers must pick off any leftover bits of meat, and clean and degrease the bones.

If you are interested in stripping your own animal bones at home for fun or profit, dermestid colony starter kits are available, assuming you don't want to pick through roadkill to gather your own. Yes, some folks like to strip deer and bear skulls for display or sale. These little carnivores can fully strip a skull in 24 hours.

What insect's specialty is poop?

That would be the dung beetle (members of the Scarabaeidae family). Poop is their life. They are masters of it. A 3-pound pile of droppings can vanish in just 2 hours, thanks to these industrious bugs. They are such specialists that certain species of dung beetle may eat the turds of only one kind of animal.

Scarab beetles have a neat little system for removing a ball of dung from a large pile. First they sort through it to separate extraneous materials like grass and worm eggs until they have pure, unadulterated poop. Then the beetle will shape and mold the dung into a perfectly smooth, round ball about the size of an apple. If this weren't amazing enough, the crazy beetle then climbs atop the dung ball and rolls it along, kind of like a log roller, by walking on top of it. This may be one of the most comical sights in the animal world. A good dung roller can move its ball some 45 feet a minute on flat ground.

Once the beetle and his dung ball reach their destination, the beetle will bury it and use it as a food source. A female dung beetle will also lay her eggs inside the ball. When the young hatch, they will have a ready supply of yummy poop to nibble on.

Not all dung beetles are "rollers"; some are known as "tunnelers." They bury their poop. Still others, known as "dwellers," just live in dung, without rolling or burying it.

They may be gross, but without dung beetles around, there would be way more poop scattered about for you to step in.

What beetle buries dead animals?

The American burying beetle (*Nicrophorus americanus*) is the undertaker of the animal world. Also known as carrion beetles, they have certainly earned their name. When they find a dead mouse or bird, they dig a hole under it and bury it.

Burying beetles can sense a dead animal from quite a distance. Several often rush to seize their prize. This results in many beetles fighting over rights to the find. The biggest male and the biggest female usually win and take joint possession.

Like any good undertaker, they prepare the corpse first. The fur or feathers are peeled away and used to line the burial chamber. The body is rolled up into a tight ball. With special glands, the beetles will spray the corpse with antimicrobial secretions from their mouth and anus. This not only preserves the carcass for future use but reduces the smell of rotting flesh that would attract competitors. These preparations can take up to 8 hours to complete.

There are mites that hitch a ride on these beetles. They hop off when the beetles bury a carcass. When maggots attack the dead animal's body, the mites proceed to feed on them.

The female beetle will lay her eggs in the dirt near the crypt. When the eggs hatch, the young will crawl into the burial hole to feed on the carcass. Mom and dad are good parents, which is rare in the insect world. They will feed their larvae by eating the rotting flesh and regurgitating it for the young. However, if there are too many larvae for the size of the carcass to feed, they will kill some off. (You can take this good parent thing only so far.)

Once widespread in the United States, the burying beetle is now an endangered species. They used to be found in at least 35 states. Now they are found in only a few Midwest states and on Block Island off of Rhode Island. Several states are trying to reintroduce them.

How long can a cockroach live with its head cut off?

Unlike us humans, who need a head for breathing, roaches do not. They breathe through spiracles found on each body segment. Oxygen is carried to each cell in the body by a set of tubes called trachea, not in blood as with mammals. No brain is needed to control breathing. Also, roaches have no blood pressure, so they can't bleed to death. Roaches don't have a brain, per se. The nervous system is spread throughout their body. Some of their brain is in the head, while the rest is scattered along the underside of the body.

About the only vital functions that would stop with decapitation are eating and drinking. But because a cockroach is cold-blooded, it can survive up to a month on one meal. Assuming the bug had a good meal before losing his head, and germs did not infect it, a roach could live 1 week without water, in a cool climate. It would, however, just kind of sit around doing nothing.

What animal mother lets her children eat her alive?

No mom of any species, including our own, has anything on the Australian social spider. Although many a spider mother protects her young by weaving a strong, protective silk around her eggs, guarding them after they are born, or gathering food for them to eat, the Australian social spider makes the supreme sacrifice—herself.

First this caring spider mother puts a protective layer of eucalyptus leaves around her newborn's nest. Then she brings back some yummy bugs for them to snack on. Soon the ungrateful spiderlings start sucking the juices out of mum's leg joints until she is unable to move anymore. Then they puke digestive juices on her and eat her alive. Talk about being a good mother.

What male spider is eaten during sex?

Contrary to popular belief, it's not the black widow. That female very rarely eats the male during copulation. The Australian female redback spider, however, eats her sexual partner 65 percent of the time. This is not that unusual, but the poor horny male redback seems to go along willingly. After the male inserts his sexual organ into the female, he flips his body over so that his abdomen is right in front of her mouth. The scrawny, little guy is only about 1 percent of her body weight, but that's OK, he still makes a nice snack. She begins to eat him almost immediately. He dutifully continues humping her until there is nothing left to hump with.

Why would he want to do such a thing? The drive to pass on one's DNA is very strong in the animal world, as it is in humans. Scientists theorize that by allowing himself to be eaten, the male redback spider gets to have sex for longer and has a better chance of completing the act. Also, the tip of the male redback's sex organ breaks off while doing it, meaning he's a one-trick pony. He gets only one chance to pass along his genes and he usually dies soon after sex anyway. So, what the heck?

Why don't they make clothes out of spider silk?

Spider silk is five times stronger than steel and 30 percent more flexible and twice as elastic as nylon. It's really great stuff. So why don't we use it for something? People have tried.

In the 1700s, French scientists figured that if the Chinese could make a fortune raising silk worms for their silk, why couldn't they raise spiders for theirs? So they put thousands of spiders into a barn and hoped to collect the silk from all their webs. The plan had one flaw—spiders are cannibals. In short order, they went from thousands of spiders to almost none. Spiders don't make good neighbors, nor do they make good lovers.

What animal's embryos are cannibals?

Somehow you don't think of embryos as being cannibalistic? But this is the case with the sand tiger shark (*Carcharias taurus*). While still in the uterus, one dominant embryo will eat the other 16 to 23 embryos and eggs. This shark has two uteri and thus gives birth to two young who took sibling rivalry to the extreme.

Why do earthworms come out on your driveway when it rains?

Earthworms have no lungs, but five hearts. Blood flowing close to the worm's skin absorbs oxygen and releases carbon dioxide directly through their cuticle (skin). They are able to survive some time in water if the oxygen content isn't too low. When the soil becomes saturated from rain, they surface to get their oxygen from the air above, which has a greater oxygen content. The wisdom of this strategy is questionable when they end up on the roadway and may never make it back underground.

Other reasons cited for the worms swimming on the sidewalks are that they come out when it rains in search of a mate, that they can travel to new areas quicker aboveground, and that when it rains there is an increase of dissolved carbon dioxide in the ground that drives up the worms. Take your pick. Regardless, it is quite disgusting when they commit mass suicide on your driveway.

Can a chicken live without a head?

Just like the cockroaches discussed earlier, it is possible for a chicken to live after having its head cut off, well most of it anyway. One famous rooster who did just fine sans head was "Mike the Headless Chicken."

Mike was 5½ months old when he gained fame. On September 10, 1945, Mike, who belonged to Fruita, Colorado, farmer Lloyd Olsen, was to be prepared for the dinner table. Olsen lopped off Mike's head with an ax, but Mike didn't seem to take notice. He kept on walking around pecking for feed. Olsen had removed most of Mike's noggin; however, a little bit of his brainstem and one ear remained. This was enough for Mike. Apparently, most of a chicken's reflex actions are controlled by the brainstem.

Seeing a good thing, Olsen spared Mike from the dinner pot and started feeding him food and water through his esophagus with an eyedropper. Mike grew and prospered. His weight went from 2½ pounds to 8 pounds over the next year and a half. Mike toured the country as "Wonder Chicken." Olsen insured Mike for $10,000 and charged folks 25 cents for a peek. Tragically, Mike choked to death after a performance in Arizona when Olsen couldn't find the eyedropper he used to keep Mike's open esophagus clear. Then Olsen barbecued Mike. (Kidding!)

Can a decapitated snake head still bite you?

Bizarre as it may sound, many people are bitten by decapitated snake heads every year. According to medical toxicologist Jeffrey Suchard at Good Samaritan Regional Medical Center in Phoenix, Arizona, 5 of the 34 snakebite victims admitted to the hospital between June 1997 and April 1998 were bitten by "dead" snakes.[3] Most victims assumed that a dead snake would be safe to pick up. Wrong! You must be very cautious for quite some time. Rattlesnake heads are dangerous for up to 90 minutes after decapitation. The biting reflex action is so strong that it needs that long to fully subside.

How dangerous are snakes in the United States?

Two families of venomous snakes are native to the United States. The vast majority are pit vipers, of the Crotalidae family, which includes copperheads, rattlesnakes, and water moccasins (cottonmouths). Pit vipers have a small pit between the eye and nostril that detects heat and allows them to better find their prey at night. They have retractable fangs that spring out when they are about to bite. Almost all poisonous snakebites in the United States are from pit vipers.

The amount of venom a person receives from a pit viper bite varies greatly. These snakes try to squirt out their venom at the exact instant that the fangs break your skin. Sometimes they misjudge the timing involved and shoot out the poison prematurely. It is not uncommon for snakebite victims to find a wet spot on their pants where the venom was squirted. Another factor affecting snakebite toxicity is size of the snake. Also, within a species, there is a wide range of venom concentrations among individual snakes.

The other family of domestic venomous snakes is Elapidae, to which the coral snake belongs. There are two species of corals—found in the southern states only. Related to the much more dangerous Asian cobras, corals have small mouths and short teeth, giving them a much less effective bite than the pit viper's. Coral snakebites are rare. "Only" about 25 people are bitten by coral snakes in the United States each year.

According to the *New England Journal of Medicine,* every state, except Hawaii, Alaska, and Maine, has at least one species of poisonous snake.[4]

What should you do if you are bitten by a venomous snake?

First off, don't make a cut in the wound and try to suck out the venom like they used to do in the old-time Western movies. This will only make the wound worse and sucking venom into your mouth isn't such a good idea anyway. Second, don't apply a tourniquet above the bite mark to prevent the venom from flowing into the rest of the body. This will completely cut off blood flow into the affected limb and may result in its loss.

So what should you do? It's pretty simple: (1) Wash the bite wound with soap and water, if available.

(2) Immobilize the bitten area and keep it lower than the heart. (3) Get medical help pronto.

If you can't get medical attention within 30 minutes, a bandage can be wrapped 2 to 4 inches above the bite to slow the venom. Unlike a tourniquet, the bandage should not cut off blood flow. It should be loose enough so that a finger can slip under it. Some commercial snakebite kits come with little rubber suction devices that you can use to suck out some of the venom. The effectiveness of this method is debatable; you still will need to see a doctor quickly.

What will a doctor do if you get a poisonous snakebite?

Depending on the species of snake that bit you and its size, the doctor may observe you for a while for adverse reactions or go right to the use of an antivenin.

There are two types of antivenin, also called antivenom. They are both derived from horse or sheep antibodies made when snake venom is injected into the animal. The derived antivenin is injected into a person's veins or muscle to neutralize the venom. The first antivenin, from a horse, was introduced to the United States in 1954. Although antivenins can reverse the effects of venom and save life and limb, they may not reverse tissue damage already done, such as necrosis. Some patients may later require skin grafts.

Are there any snakes big enough to swallow a person whole?

There are some pretty darn big snakes out there. The longest snakes are pythons, which can reach up to 30 feet. The heaviest snakes are the anacondas, which can weigh in at 235 pounds. These big boys are capable of downing some big chow (not the dog, although they could). The biggest snake meal on record is that of an African rock python that swallowed a 130-pound antelope whole.

The thing about eating a large serving of food is that it takes a long time to digest. This presents a problem because food begins to rot if it stays in a snake too long. This makes for the production of noxious gases. To avoid a bad case of indigestion, snakes frequently barf up partially digested meals.

In answer to the question, in very rare cases, snakes have been reported to have swallowed children or small adults.[5] There's a reason snakes that are large enough to eat people don't. It's not because we taste bad but a simple matter of practicality. Snakes begin swallowing their food from the head end and work their way down. In the case of humans, the snake encounters a tough obstacle when it reaches the shoulders. While snakes can ingest some very large animals, they usually choose ones that have more gradual contours, like an alligator. If a careless serpent tries to swallow something too large, it can choke to death.

What animal sticks its stomach out of its mouth to feed?

If you guessed sea star, you were really paying attention in high school bio class after all. Stars love clams. However, a clam can be a tough nut to crack. So the stars wrap their five sucker-studded arms around the clam and pull the two shell halves apart just enough to invert their stomachs through their mouths right into the clam. Once inside, the stomach secretes digestive juices to liquefy the clam's body, which is then sucked back into the star's mouth with its stomach.

Do some animals have a bone in their penis?

Yes, almost all mammals have a bone in their member. The only ones who don't are humans, hyenas, marsupials, members of the horse family, and members of the rabbit family. All other mammals have a baculum, also known as an os penis or penis bone. (This is where the slang word for erection—boner—comes from.) The word is Latin for "stick" or "staff." The baculum is used to stiffen the mammalian penis during copulation. We humans don't need one because a man achieves an erection through the power of hydraulics—that is, blood flow engorging the penis. In case you are wondering, some animals have very long bacula. The walrus can have a penis bone of some 21 inches.

It is interesting that there is an analogous bone in the mammalian female, called the baubellum or *os clitoridis,* which is also missing in humans.

That's not all that gross, is it? Well, how about this? The male raccoon has a penis bone that has been put to practical use by humans (see page 100).

How does a mother kangaroo keep her pouch clean?

The mother-to-be kangaroo begins cleaning her pouch several days before the arrival of the little joey. That's what a baby roo is called. When it's time, the blind, peanut-size little fella must make the trip from the birth canal into the pouch unassisted by mom, clawing its way upward through her fur. This arduous journey takes about 15 minutes. Once inside the pouch, the joey will latch on to one of four teats and suckle at the same one until it is weaned.

A couple of days after giving birth, the mother will mate again, and the resulting embryo will remain dormant inside her until the joey either leaves or dies in the pouch, at which time it will develop to replace the departed offspring. This unique feature of kangaroo reproduction is known as embryonic diapause.

The joey stays in the pouch for 8 to 10 months, after which time it takes short forays into the outside world, returning often to nurse, until it is about a year old.

A kangaroo has one of the longest tongues, relative to body size, in the animal kingdom, which mom uses to clean her joey and her pouch. She essentially licks the excrement out.

Additionally, a mother kangaroo can control the muscles of her pouch to regulate its size and the size of the opening. By contracting her muscles, she can secure her joey so it doesn't go flying out as she is bounding across the Outback—nature's version of the car seat.

Who makes purses from kangaroo scrotums?

You guessed it—the Aborigines. This is no joke. The Aborigines have a legend explaining how this practice came to be. They believe that there once lived an aboriginal boy in central Australia. One day he came upon a small kangaroo in the bush, caught it by the tail, and made a purse out of its scrotum. He gave it to his girlfriend, and she kept seeds and berries in it. Next he saw a large kangaroo. He caught it with a spear and made another purse from its thick "pouch." He gave it to his father, who kept stones and things of value in it.

Ever since then, male kangaroo scrotum purses have been popular among the Aborigines. A soft pliable one for the women, a strong wrinkled one for the men. They became important as a man's own symbol of masculinity and were recognized as bringing good luck. Today, they are known as lucky bags or pouches.

You can actually buy kangaroo scrotum pouches

online for between $10 and $25, depending on size. They are advertised as a romantic or sentimental present, perfect for weddings, birthdays, Christmas, or as a very special corporate gift. The sellers suggest hanging one from your rearview mirror, or from your back bumper, if you are a guy.

To those of you who are alarmed about the killing of poor innocent kangaroos for their scrotal sacs, it may ease your concerns to know that the roo is protected by the Australian government. Only enough animals are harvested to keep their population under control. So, go ahead and get one to hang from your Christmas tree.

Is a dog's mouth cleaner than your mouth?

Yes, and no. It's a common belief among the uninformed that a dog's mouth is cleaner than a human's. Although there are some truly dirty humans out there, most of us don't eat garbage, dead animals, or our own poop. These rather distasteful practices would make the dog mouth dirtier than your own. However, assuming the dog in question hasn't been licking his butt or nibbling on a dead critter, his mouth may have less harmful germs than that of a fellow human being. This is because dogs tend to have dog germs and people have people germs. Their germs are species specific—that is, they harm dogs, not people. As a rule, we don't get dog illnesses and they don't get ours. So their mouths may be "cleaner." Regardless, you'd still probably be better off French kissing a person than a poodle.

What is the most dangerous breed of dog?

It certainly isn't the golden retriever, which may be the world's mushiest dog. When it comes to being just plain mean and aggressive, there are a few breeds that stand out. They are, as you might guess, the usual suspects: the Rottweiler and the pit bull (big surprise). Pit bulls make up only about 2 percent of the dog population but account for 50 percent of serious attacks. It is estimated that 1 pit bull in 55 will seriously bite a person during any given year. And 1 in 16 pit bull bites will result in serious injury, whereas the ratios for German shepherds are 1 in 156 and for Dobermans 1 in 296.

How can you avoid being bitten by a dog? Experts advise avoiding dogs that are chained, eating, sleeping, playing with a toy, unaltered, and/or male and stay away from pit bulls, Rottweilers, German shepherds, Dobermans . . . maybe you should just avoid dogs altogether.

When was the maiming of cats common?

During the Middle Ages, many viewed cats as evil. They were furtive, nocturnal, and thought to be supernatural servants of witches. Cats were stealthy, elusive, and their eyes glowed at night. Obviously, they possessed dark powers. These superstitions led to some abuse of cats and a general decline in their population.

The maiming of cats was thought to protect one from evil, and cats figured prominently in some Middle Age cures. If you had an upset stomach, it was said that a few plops of cat poop in your wine was just the thing (Dark Age Pepto-Bismol). A little blood from a cat's ear was great for warding off the flu or pneumonia. Sucking the blood out of a severed cat's tail was believed to relieve pains.

By the 1300s, cat numbers had fallen and rat populations had risen dramatically. Some scholars say this led to the speed with which the Black Death (carried by the fleas on rats) swept through Europe.

When were cat mummies used as fertilizer?

The ancient Egyptians mummified all kinds of animals—apes, bulls, dogs, hawks, snakes, the odd hippo—but were especially fond of cats. Around 900 BCE, Egyptian religious beliefs held that cats were the living embodiment of the goddess Bast (also spelled Bastet). She had the body of a woman and the head of a cat. The sacred cat was highly revered and cats were raised by the thousands in and around temples devoted to Bast. It was illegal to kill a cat, punishable by death. Dead cats were mummified, as were mice to keep them company in the afterlife.

Between 332 and 30 BCE, the fortunes of the kitties changed. They were raised for the specific purpose of mummification. People bought them on their way to the temples and left them as an offering. Apparently, 2- to 4-month-old kittens were favored for mummies, probably because they more easily fit into the mummy container. Autopsies show that most had their necks broken.

Dead cats were mummified and buried in huge mass graves. Archaeologists estimate the numbers to be well into the millions. In 1888, a railway company laying new track came upon a mass burial ground containing hundreds of thousands of cat mummies. Seeing the potential for profit, they were pulverized and sent back to England as fertilizer. Thousands more were used as fuel for the company's locomotives.

What disease can you get from your cat?

There's a disease that only your cat can give you and that affects more than 60 million Americans. It's caused by a one-celled protozoan named *Toxoplasma gondii*. Most infected people never realize they have it because their immune systems keep the organism from causing symptoms. Pregnant women and those with a compromised immune system, however, should beware.

Toxoplasma is found in cat feces. By accidentally swallowing cat poop, either after handling the litter box or touching contaminated soil in the garden, you can become infected. Raw meats such as pork, lamb, and venison also harbor these protozoa.

Pregnant women who first come in contact with

Toxoplasma just before becoming or while pregnant can infect their baby. Blood tests are routinely done on pregnant women to see if they've ever been infected in their life. If so, there is no need to worry. If not, the woman will be advised to avoid cat feces at all costs. Some concerned mothers-to-be send Fluffy away until after they give birth. Babies born with *Toxoplasma* may have serious eye or brain damage.

Cats become infected by going outside and fraternizing with other cats, or by eating infected prey or raw meat. You can also get it from raw and undercooked meats. To protect yourself if you are pregnant, keep your cat indoors and feed it only dry or canned cat food. Also, wear protective gloves when changing the litter box or gardening. Better yet, have another person change the litter for you—every day. Happily, your cat will stay infected only for a few weeks, so by following these guidelines you should be OK.

Why do cats like to rub up against you?

You cat people out there will say it's because Fluffy loves you sooo much. Although this may or may not be true, cats rub on people for the same reason wild big cats rub on trees—to mark their territory.

House cats have glands around their forehead, mouth, and chin that release pheromones. These are chemicals that mammals use to communicate with other animals. When a cat rubs its face on your legs or your furniture it is spreading scents telling other cats to stay away: You and your house are taken.

Why are they breeding bald chickens?

Israel is hot. So Israeli chicken farmers need to keep their birds cool. In lieu of expensive air-conditioning systems, ever-resourceful animal breeders have found a better way—bald chickens.

These creatures are quite hideous. Through the miracle of cross-breeding, scientists at Hebrew University have come up with a completely bald chicken. Not only are these normal-size birds less fatty they are also pre-plucked, saving even more money.

How is bull sperm collected?

Bulls are like stallions. When one is found with the desirable traits that breeders look for, its sperm can become quite valuable. Champion bulls have their sperm collected so that the best meat-producing animal can be bred. How does one collect bull sperm? The process isn't pretty, but here goes:

The bull must first be "stimulated" (use your imagination); then it is presented with a steer (castrated male) to mount. This prevents accidental penetration of a cow and the loss of sperm. As the randy bull tries in vain to mount the steer, some poor technician must run over to the bull with a container, put it over the bull's penis, and get him to ejaculate into it. Happily, the whole thing is over in the blink of an eye, about 2 seconds.

A champion bull can make its owner up to $125,000, and he will end up siring some 100,000 offspring from his sperm. Bulls are selected for sperm donation by the size of their balls. At 1 year of age, bulls have their balls measured. Bulls that have testicles that measure more than 30 centimeters in circumference are selected. Only 1 in 100 bulls meets this criterion. The other 99 percent are shipped off to the slaughterhouse. The big boys are spared and can expect regular servicing.

Breeders use computers to help them analyze the genetic makeup of all cattle. This information is entered into a database, which is then used to select the parents with the best traits to breed tomorrow's super-cows.

How do they inseminate racehorses?

Natural, or hand, breeding is the most commonly used reproductive technique for racehorses. A compliant mare is allowed to stand on a level surface that has good traction and is free of physical barriers. If she is receptive, she will hunch her back with hind legs spread, and pelvis tipped down. Less compliant mares may be restrained to prevent kicking and injury to the stallion.

The mare's tail is bandaged and her vulva washed with water and a mild soap solution. The stallion may first be introduced to a "fluff" mare, whose only purpose is to excite him. Once he achieves an erection, the fluff mare is removed and his penis is also washed. He then may slowly approach and mount the mare. Ejaculation occurs quickly, and he returns to his life of leisure until his services are next required. All in all, not a bad deal.

Thoroughbred sires can earn their owners a fortune, much more than they make on the track. The top stallion in this regard was named Storm Cat. He was a descendant of Triple Crown winner Secretariat. Storm Cat's offspring have earned more than $90 million at the racetrack. As such, he could fetch up to $500,000 per mating session with a mare. He made over $20 million for stud fees in 1 year alone!

How are horses artificially inseminated?

Lately, some horses are being bred by artificial insemination. The stallion's semen must first be collected. As with the live insemination just described, a "fluff" mare is used to stimulate him. When he is good and excited, he is made to mount a padded dummy mare that has an artificial vagina, called a boot. A handler then holds his penis in the boot and collects his sperm. (Yuck!) Once collected, the semen can be split into about a dozen portions and chilled or frozen.

The insemination of the mare is another unsavory affair. Her privates are washed and her tail bandaged. Then comes the gross part. A technician wearing a well-lubricated rubber glove that extends up to the elbow must put a plunger syringe all the way into the mare's vagina and through the cervix and squirt the semen into the uterus. (Not a job for the squeamish.)

What is a Judas goat?

Judas goats are the traitors of the animal world. They are goats that are trained to "befriend" other animals and lead them to their doom. Slaughterhouses use goats that are trained to associate with sheep and cattle and then lead them to pens or the bolt gun. The Judas goat's life is spared. They are also used to help round up feral goats that are marked for eradication.

How do they sex chickens?

There are people called "chicken sexers." Their job is to separate the female chicks from the male chicks. Sounds easy, right? Well, this is a highly specialized profession that only a handful of folks, predominantly Japanese (the art of chicken sexing originated in Japan) who have been taught the art from a young age, have mastered. You see, chicks don't have any external sex organs to look at. These experts, who make in the range of $60,000 to $70,000 a year, can sex around 1,000 birds an hour. How do they do it? By literally squeezing the feces out of the birds. This opens up the rectum and allows the sexer to look for a small bump. Chicks with the bump are roosters; bumpless chicks are hens.

Why do they have to sex a chick? Because on an egg farm, roosters are not needed, except for the odd stud bird. The male chicks are destroyed immediately.

Have you ever worn whale vomit?

You'd never know if you did. It's called ambergris, and it is used in perfumes and fixatives and, yes, it's regurgitated by sperm whales.

When a sperm whale swallows something that is too hard or sharp to digest, like a giant squid's beak, its intestines secrete a fatty bile to coat the object, facilitating its passage through the beast. Whales expel lumps of this stuff from time to time that can range in size from a couple of ounces to over 100 pounds. When first expelled or removed from the whale, this preambergris is pale white, soft, and smells like feces. After a few years of exposure to the water, salt, and sun, it becomes a hard, dark, waxy blob with a sweet, earthy, animal-like aroma. Experts describe its odor as like isopropyl alcohol, only richer, smoother, and without the stinging harshness.

Ambergris is quite valuable and can be found floating around in the oceans or washed up on the beach. Raw ambergris sells for around $10 a gram, although high-quality samples are worth much more. A 32-pound lump of the stuff recently washed up on a beach in Australia and fetched a whopping $750,000!

Due to its high cost and lack of a consistently reliable

supply, synthetic versions now exist, but higher-end perfumes may still contain the real thing.

Are there fish scales in your lipstick?

The cosmetics companies have very few restrictions on what ingredients they may put in their products. Lipstick, for instance, has many ingredients; some may surprise or even disgust you. The main ingredients in lipstick are waxes, fats and oils, emollients, and pigments. A quick outline of each will be instructive:

- Wax makes the lipstick easy to apply and helps it hold its shape in the tube. Some of the waxes include beeswax from honeycombs, carnauba wax from the leaves of the Brazilian wax palm tree, and candelilla wax from the Mexican carnauba plant.
- Fats and oils in lipstick include cocoa butter, lanolin, petrolatum, mineral oil, olive oil, and castor oil. An ingredient like castor oil provides a durable, shiny film.
- Moisturizers and other ingredients like aloe vera, amino acids, collagen (protein from the connective tissue of young cows), and vitamin E help keep the lips soft and supple.
- Pigments include various red and orange dyes that are mixed with titanium white to achieve a wide range of colors.

Lipsticks are made a lot like crayons. The other ingredients are ground up and mixed together with wax, oil, and lanolin. The mixture is heated and stirred often and pored into a mold. A quick blast of heat gives the stick its final, glossy finish.

Finally, yes, fish scales have been used over the years in lipsticks and nail polishes for their shimmering qualities. Known as "pearl essence," these ground up fish scales commonly come from herring. According to the National Marine Fisheries Service, pearl essence from herring and other fish is still used in the manufacture of lipstick and nail polish.[6] However, new synthetic versions are now available.

Are there cow brains and crushed bugs in your makeup?

If you find the idea of rubbing ground up fish scales on your lips unsettling, you are gonna love this. The cosmetics industry has some other gross surprises in their products.

Some skin-care products contain cerebrosides. These glycolipids are used to promote smoother, moister skin. Sounds nice, but what is this stuff? Well, the raw material for cerebrosides comes from cow brains and other nervous-system tissue from cattle, oxen, and pigs.

Many cosmetics also use carmine, carminic acid, or cochineal—all pigments derived from crushed cochineal insects, as a red colorant. The red color is obtained by crushing the bodies of female insects, such as *Dacty-*

lopius coccus, containing eggs and larvae. (How pleasant.) These soft-bodied, flat, oval, wooly insects live on *Opuntia* cacti in the Canary Islands and Central and South America, and they use carminic acid as a defense against predators. Harvesting the insects is done by hand and is quite labor-intensive. About 155,000 bugs are needed to make 1 kilogram of cochineal dye.

Carmine is one of the few colorants deemed safe enough for use in eye makeup. It's also found in lipstick, rouge, blush, and hair and skin products. Because it is more light and heat stable than many of the synthetic colorants, it's used in meats (which must be labeled such in the United States), dairy products, baked goods, jams and preserves, surimi, alcoholic beverages, juices, pie fillings, and gelatins. Cochineal, however, is forbidden in kosher foods. You probably consume only a few drops of this stuff in a year's time.

What aphrodisiac is made from beetle wings?

It's called "Spanish fly," but it's made from the dried wings of South American meloid beetles. Spanish fly has been used by native peoples for a couple of thousand years. Its active ingredient is cantharidin, a chemical that, in addition to making you nauseous, also gives you a long-lasting, painful erection and a wicked itch in the urinary tract. They say the best way to relieve the itch is to ejaculate. Proper dosage was a problem with Spanish fly—too much could damage the kidneys, cause convulsions, or even death. This may explain why it sort of fell out of favor in the 1800s.

Where do people lick toads to get high?

The lengths to which some people will go to take a hallucinogenic trip! There's a certain amphibian found in the American Southwest known as the Colorado River toad and the Sonoran Desert toad (*Bufo alvarius*). This particular toad has a unique method of deterring predators—it secretes a milky venom containing a combination of two powerful drugs—dimethyltryptamine and bufotenine—both of which are hallucinogenic.

Some folks, nature lovers presumably, collect the toad's milky secretions by stroking the toad under the chin, causing it to exude its venom. Once collected, the milky venom is dried and smoked for a "natural" high. By smoking the venom, users are protected from the poisons it contains, which are not volatile on heating.

According to the Arizona Department of Fish and Game, some more adventurous souls prefer a different, more dangerous way to go on a toad trip.[7] They lick the venom directly from the toad's skin. Bufotenine is classified as a psychoactive drug under Arizona law. By licking the toads, users are not only ingesting bufotenine, but also the poisons found in the venom, running the risk of severe illness or death. But what the heck, a high's a high.

Cane toads can also be licked for a high, in case you were wondering.

What people were paid to eat toads?

The modern-day term *toady* comes from the toad-eaters who worked at fairs in seventeenth- and eighteenth-century England. Toad-eaters would travel from fair to fair and market to market with a snake oil salesman, who peddled bogus cure-alls to the masses.

The toady was an underpaid hireling who—in front of a gullible crowd—swallowed live toads (thought at the time to be poisonous). The toady would fall to the ground as if very ill. The quack salesman would then produce a bottle of magical cure-all and pour some down the "dying" toady's throat and affect a miraculous cure. The duly impressed crowd would snatch up vials of this wonderful elixir.

What flowers are pollinated by carrion flies?

The purpose of lovely, fragrant flowers is not to please people but to attract insects and other animals to promote pollination. Most flowers look and smell very nice to us humans, and pollinators. There's one flower that targets a small niche of potential pollinators—carrion flies. These flies love rotting meat and this is what the corpse flower (*Rafflesia arnoldii*) smells like. It is quite the most unusual flower in the world. It is a parasite that has no leaves, stem, or true roots. It sends feeding tubes into its host's tissue. The only part of the plant that is visible is its up to 3-foot-wide brown flower—the largest flower in the world, which can weigh up to 115 pounds! It grows only on certain vines in the islands of Southeast Asia. Not only do the brown flowers resemble rotting meat but they smell like it—and profoundly so.

Another stinky species, nicknamed "corpse flower," is the Indonesian titan arum, or *Amorphophallus titanum*. It has a cluster of flowers that can weigh 170 pounds, reach up to a height of 12 feet, and is shaped like an erect phallus, as you can guess from its genus name.

A stinky plant that you may be familiar with is the maidenhair tree (*Ginkgo biloba*). The Ginkgo is best known as a "living fossil," being the sole survivor of an ancient family of plants that went extinct 200 million years ago. It was long thought extinct by Western scientists. Considered a sacred tree, it was kept alive by Buddhist priests on temple grounds in China, Japan, and Korea. The tree found its way to America in 1784. Today, only the male trees are widely planted because the female's fruits have a stomach-turning stench like that of puke or rancid butter, once they fall from the tree. If you haven't heard of the tree, you may have heard of its main by-product—Ginkgo extract, which is obtained from its leaves and is said to improve memory. It is added to some energy drinks.

When did gentlemen write love poems about their sweetheart's fleas?

For most of human history, being infested with bugs was an accepted part of life. Although the other primates may groom each other by removing parasites, we humans don't. However, some seventeenth-century Frenchmen would take a flea from their lover and keep it in a tiny gold box hung around their neck, where it could feed daily on their blood. Now, that's love!

Who kept naked slaves covered in honey to catch flies?

Legend has it that in ancient Egypt, the wealthy paid flea catchers to come to their homes. How did they catch fleas? They covered themselves in milk and stood in the middle of the room. After a while the fleas were said to have all landed on the flea catcher, who would then leave with the bugs. Egyptian King Pepi II similarly is rumored to have kept near him naked slaves covered in honey to keep flies from annoying him.

European women had another method of catching fleas. They wore animal furs around their necks covered in sticky tree sap that would trap the little vermin. This practice later led to the wearing of fur stoles and boas purely for fashion.

Can you make a mosquito explode by stretching your skin taut?

The scientific literature on this subject is a little thin. There are numerous apocryphal accounts that this phenomenon is legit. The story goes like this: If you pull your skin taut near a mosquito who is feeding on you, its proboscis will get stuck. The mosquito's anticoagulants will keep on working and blood will continue to enter the skeeter until it bursts. Everyone seems to agree that you can trap the mosquito this way. There are conflicting reports on the exploding part. This is one of those urban legends that you will need to go out into the backyard this summer and try out for yourself, if you're a 12-year-old boy that is.

Scientists, however, *are* able to make mosquitoes explode in the laboratory. When a mosquito gets full, a chemical is released that tells it to stop feeding. By disabling that chemical signal, scientists can make the little suckers feed until they burst. Must be quite a disgusting sight to behold.

ENDNOTES

Deliciously Disgusting: Gross Foods

1. Josephine Ma, "Guangdong Gourmets Eat 10,000 Cats a Day," *South China Morning Post*, December 4, 2002, available at www.scmp.com/portal/site/SCMP (accessed May 10, 2007).

2. Anthony Bourdain, "Not for Vegetarians . . . Cobra Heart" [video clip], 28 sec, available at www.youtube.com/watch?v=ovwj0FYN0Qg (accessed November 2007).

3. Anthony Bourdain, "Fetal Duck Egg (Balut)" [video clip], 45 sec, available at www.youtube.com/watch?v=RXucin9iIaE&feature=related (accessed November 2007).

4. K. C. Chan, "Eat Live Monkey Brains! In Pingxiang, Guangxi, It Really Exists!," *Daily Apple,* October 21, 1998, available at http://maxent.org/ch/monkey_brains_ad.html (accessed May 30, 2007).

5. U.S. Food and Drug Administration Center for Food Safety and Applied Nutrition, *Defect Action Level Handbook*, rev. ed., May 1998, available at www.cfsan.fda.gov/~dms/dalbook.html (accessed April 21, 2007).

6. Ohio State University, "Insects as Human Food," available at www.ohioonline.osu.edu/hyg-fact/2000/2160.html (accessed February 8, 2007).

7. H. B. Wainwright, W. L. Heyward, J. P. Middaugh, C. L. Hatheway, A. P. Harpster, and T. R. Bender, "Food-Borne Botulism in Alaska, 1947–1985: Epidemiology and Clinical Findings," *Journal of Infectious Disease* 157 (1988): 1158–1162.

8. "On the Menu Today: Horse Penis and Testicles with Chili Dip," *China Daily*, available at www.chinadaily.com.cn/english/doc/2006-02/17/content_521375.htm (accessed April 4, 2007).

Creepy Crawlies: Bugs and Worms

1. S. Scrivener, H. Yemaneberhan, M. Zebenigus, D. Tilahun, S. Girma, S. Ali, P. McElroy, A. Custovic, A. Woodcock, D. Pritchard, A. Venn, and J. Britton, "Independent Effects of Intestinal Parasite Infection and Domestic Allergen Exposure on Risk of Wheeze in Ethiopia: A Nested Case-Control Study," *The Lancet* 358, no. 9292 (2001): 1493–1499.

2. R. W. Summer, D. E. Elliott, J. F. Urban, R. Thompson, and J. V. Weinstock, "*Trichus suis* Therapy in Crohn's Disease," *Gut* 54 (2005): 87–90.

Teeny Meanies: Germs

1. T. W. Pope, P. T. Ender, W. K. Woelk, M. A. Koroscil, T. M. Koroscil, "Bacterial Contamination of Paper Currency," *Southern Medical Journal* 95, no. 12 (2002): 1408–1410.

2. Patricia Gadsby, "Filthy Lucre—Money Is Contaminated with Bacteria," *Discover*, October 1998, pp. 78–84.

3. Malcolm W. Browne, "Drug Money (in the literal sense) Is a New Legal Twist," *New York Times*, September 23, 1997, p. F5.

4. C. P. Gerba, C. Wallis, and J. L. Melnick, "Microbial Hazards of Household Toilets: Droplet Production and the Fate of Residual Organisms," *Applied Microbiology* 30 (1975): 229–237.

5. Ibid.

6. The Clorox Company, "Office Germs Research 2006 Results," news release, February 16, 2006.

7. Ibid.

8. Sheri L. Maxwell and Charles P. Gerba, personal communication, August 20, 2007.

9. K. A. Reynolds, P. M. Watt, S. A. Boone, and C. P. Gerba, "Occurrence of Bacteria and Biochemical Markers on Public Surfaces," *International Journal of Environmental Health Research* 15 (2005): 225–234.

10. Ibid.

11. Joan Verdon, "What's on a Shopping Cart Handle?," *The (Bergen County) Record*, September 30, 2005, p. B4.

12. Hugh Morley, "Wiping Away Grocery Cart Health Hazards," *The (Bergen County) Record*, April 4, 2007, p. B3.

13. Kristy Steves, *News at Five*, Fox Network, Cleveland, Ohio, May 3, 2006.

14. M. Ryan, R. Christian, and J. Wohlrabe, "Handwashing and Respiratory Illness Among Young Adults in Military Training," *American Journal of Preventive Medicine* 21 (2001): 79–83.

15. American Society for Microbiology and the Soap and Detergent Manufacturers Association, press conference, Washington, DC, September 21, 2005.

Cleanliness Is Next to Godliness: Hygiene

1. Jay Stuller, "Cleanliness Has Only Recently Become a Virtue," *Smithsonian* (February 1991): 126–135.

2. G. L. Simons, *The Illustrated Book of Sexual Records.* New York: Random House, 1987.

3. *Guinness World Records*, New York: Bantam, 2007.

Taking Care of "Business": Feces

1. B. A. Sikirov, "Cardio-Vascular Events at Defecation: Are They Avoidable?," *Medical Hypotheses* 32, no. 3 (1990): 231–233.

2. K. W. Heaton, "Detection of Pseudodiarrhea by Simple Clinical Assessment of Intestinal Transit Rate," *British Medical Journal* 300 (1990): 439–440.

3. D. F. Altomare and V. Memeo, "Colonic Explosion During Diathermy Colostomy," *Diseases of the Colon and Rectum* 36 (1993): 291–292.

4. University of Iowa, "Fire Safety in the Operating Room," available at www.uiowa.edu/~medtest/reference/FIREsafety.pdf (accessed August 22, 2007).

Sweat, Spit, and Spew: Bodily Fluids

1. Trevor Cox, "The Hunt for the Worst Sound in the World," available at www.acoustics.salford.ac.uk/news2.htm (accessed February 15, 2007).

2. Robert Matthews, "I've Lost My Appetite . . . ," *New Scientist* 2255 (2000): 7.

3. Emetophobia, "Frequently Asked Questions about Vomiting," available at http://faq.emetophobia.net/vomiting.html (accessed February 10, 2007).

Body Oddities

1. Francis M. Fesmire, "Termination of Intractable Hiccups with Digital Rectal Massage," *Annals of Emergency Medicine* 17, no. 8 (1988): 872.

2. *Guinness World Records 2004*, London: Guinness Publishing, 2004.

3. A. Park, "The Case of the Disappearing Leech," *British Journal of Plastic Surgery* 46 (1993): 543.

4. ABC Science Online, "The Great Belly Button Lint Survey: The Results," available at www.abc.net.au/science/k2/lint/results .htm (accessed February 9, 2007).

5. *Guinness World Records 2002*, London: Guinness Publishing, 2002.

6. J. A. Heathcote, "Why Do Old Men Have Big Ears?," *British Medical Journal* 311 (1995): 1668; and Y. Asai, M. Yoshimura, N. Nago, and T. Yamada, "Correlation of Ear Length with Age in Japan," *British Medical Journal* 312 (1996): 582.

7. D. McLean, R. G. Forsythe, and I. A. Kapkin, "Unusual Side Effects of Clomipramine Associated with Yawning," *Canadian Journal of Psychiatry* 28 (1983): 569–570.

Victoria's Secrets: The Female Body

1. Jack Hanna, interview by Larry King, *Larry King Live*, CNN, September 1, 2006.

2. B. M. Randall, R. P. Vance, and T. H. McCalmont, "Xenolingual Autoeroticism," *American Journal of Forensic Medicine and Pathology* 11 (1990): 89–92.

Members Only: The Male Body

1. "Russian Museum to Exhibit Rasputin's Penis," available at

www.mosnews.com/news/2004/04/28/rasputin.shtml (accessed March 10, 2007).

Death and Beyond

1. "Keith Richards Says He Snorted Father's Ashes," available at www.msnbc.msn.com/id/17933669 (accessed April 5, 2007).
2. Robert McFadden, "They Said She Was D.O.A., But Then the Body Bag Moved," *New York Times*, November 18, 1994, p. B7.
3. Ed Friedlander, "Autopsy," available at www.pathguy.com /autopsy.htm (accessed March 20, 2007).

Fish and Foul: Animals

1. B. Wilson, R. S. Batty, and L. M. Dill, "Pacific and Atlantic Herring Produce Burst Pulse Sounds," *Proceedings of the Royal Society B: Biological Sciences* 271 (2003, Suppl. 3): S95–S97.
2. Robert Kenney, "Hagfish: The Most Disgusting Creature in the Sea," paper presented at Friends of Oceanography Lecture Series, University of Rhode Island, Narragansett, Rhode Island, March 25, 2002.
3. Thomas Ropp, "Dead Snakes Still Bite," *The Arizona Republic*, June 25, 1999, p. A1.
4. B. S. Gold, R. C. Dart, and R. A. Barish, "Bites of Venomous Snakes," *New England Journal of Medicine* 347, no. 5 (2002): 347–356.
5. Nutan Shukla, "Strange World of Snakes," available at www .tribuneindia.com.2001/20011209/spectrum/nature.htm (accessed March 10, 2007).
6. National Oceanic and Atmospheric Administration, National Marine Fisheries Service, Northeast Fisheries Center, "What Is Pearl Essence?," available at www.nefsc.noaa.gov/faq/fish faq2b1.html (accessed April 2, 2007).
7. Gene Sloan, "Arizona Says People Step One Toad Over the Line," *USA Today*, August 4, 1994, p. A1.

ABOUT THE AUTHOR

This is the sixth book of trivial knowledge by **Don Voorhees** (and definitely the most disgusting!). He lives quietly with his wonderful wife, Lisa, and their two children, Eric and Dana, in northeastern Pennsylvania.